D1116622

Pets in Therapy

Pets in Therapy

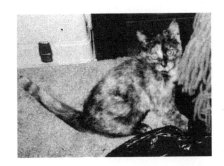
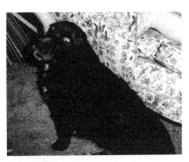

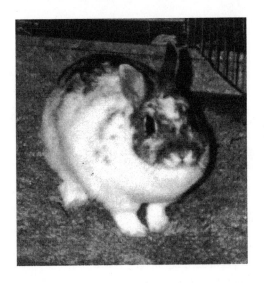

edited by

*Margaret N. Abdill, CPN, ADC
& Denise Juppé*

Published and distributed by

Idyll Arbor, Inc.

PO Box 720, Ravensdale, WA 98051 (425) 432-3231

Library of Congress Cataloguing-in-Publication Data
Pets in therapy / edited by Margaret Abdil & Denise Juppé.
    p. cm.
    "Earlier edition published by Geriatric Educational Consultants (1992) under the title Pets and older people: a guide for pet therapy programs."
    Rev. ed. of: Pets and older people. 1992.
    Includes bibliographical references (p.) and index.
    ISBN 1-882883-29-2 (alk. paper)
    1. Pets -- Therapeutic use.   I. Abdil. Margaret, 1947-   . II. Juppé, Denise. 1950-   . III. Pets and older people.
RM931.A65P495 1997
615.8'515--dc21   97-16973

ISBN 1-882883-29-2

Acknowledgments

In writing these acknowledgments I have come to realize just how many people have touched my life as I have worked to implement pet therapy.

First, I thank my husband, Firman, for his love and support, not only while I was preparing this manual but through twenty some-odd years of sharing our lives together. He has also been a constant support in caring for our "boys" and has been *most* helpful in keeping up with our family's growth from one dog to four!

At work, I owe special thanks to Pat Hirschlein, who has been my wonderful secretary and support person for our pet therapy program, cheerfully putting up first with Bandit's antics and now Prancer's need for constant attention and affection. Pat Mitchell, my Woodworking advisor, has integrated pet therapy into her responsibilities and has been constant in her efforts to provide structured pet visits. I also thank my supervisors, Tammy George and Maria Mattera, who implement my programming on a daily basis and who have been very supportive in integrating our pet therapy program throughout the facility.

I would also like to give thanks and acknowledgment to the following people:

To Rick Small, Administrator, and Barbara Fels, Associate Administrator, both of the Masonic Home of New Jersey, who have supported the pet therapy program at my facility.

To the Willingboro Veterinary Clinic, PA in Willingboro, New Jersey. They are further cited in the dedication of this manual.

To the breeders I have worked with so closely. Ron Howard, who has since passed away, showed me how to train Bandit and taught me many invaluable dog handling skills. I will always remember his voice on the telephone calling my office to ask, "Is Bandit there?" And to Jackie and Jerry Pentel of Golden Haven Golden Retrievers in Denton, Maryland who have been so supportive and caring, and who nurture their puppies from birth on, to make them the great "people dogs" that they are.

To the Brandy Lane Dog Training School and its trainers, particularly Nancy Bratyon. Her advice and expertise over our years of dog handling are greatly appreciated. She has always been available to answer questions and to help in any way necessary.

To my special friend, Beverly Haaf, author of "No More Mr. Nice Guy" – a romance novel about an Activity Director and her therapy dog. She not only made people aware of the Activity Profession, she also gave *me* the opportunity to make people aware of pet therapy and its benefits as we traveled together to civic groups and book signings.

It would be an oversight to not mention my dear cousin, Karla Pullen, who has been like the daughter we never had. We've held her in our arms as an infant, enjoyed her childhood years and now are so proud of her as she fulfills her job responsibilities as an administrative secretary in our facility. She has retyped the second edition of this manual for me. She is also our "dog sitter" when we occasionally go on vacation.

To Ricki Cunninghis of Geriatric Educational Consultants, educator, consultant and author, who first encouraged me to put on paper what I have learned in implementing pet therapy, so as to be able to share it with others.

To joan burlingame and Idyll Arbor, Inc. who will publish this newly updated version of "Pets in Therapy" (previously entitled "Pets and Older People.").

Finally, to Phil Arkow, Chair of the Latham Foundation Child and Animal Abuse Prevention Program, nationally known humane educator, author and lecturer on human-companion animal bonding and animal assisted therapy and to Harriet Doolittle, VMD, Program Coordinator for the Animal Science Department at Camden Co. College. Together they created and taught a basic and advanced course on Animal-Assisted Activities and Animal-Assisted Therapy. Participating in both of their classes has given me a wealth of information and a much deeper understanding of the human-animal bond.

Dedication

This manual is dedicated to the doctors and staff at the Willingboro Veterinary Clinic, Willingboro, New Jersey. Their initial help in selecting books, breeds, breeders and trainers to assist in developing my program was invaluable.

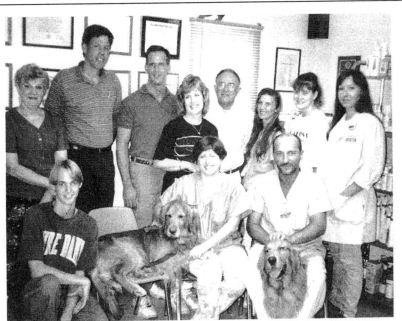

The Willingboro Veterinary Clinic. Pictured (left to right): Front row — Wayne Conrey, "Tidewater's Golden Prancer," Amy Mendelson, VMD, Jim Lippincott, "Nicholas John Firman" (Woodshop dog). Second row — Connie Anderson, Lawrence H. Wolf, VMD, Michael G. Torline, DVM, Cindy LeConey, Samuel Longer, DVM, Terry Craythorn, Chris Murphy, Linda Schiavo.

Samuel Longer, DVM (recently deceased), Lawrence Wolf, VMD and Phyllis Kimmelman, DVM were already a part of the clinic when my program was just in the talking stage. They have since been joined by Amy Mendelson, VMD and Michael Torline, DVM. Each of these doctors has played an important part in the care of our pets (And their "parents" — I might add!) Both doctors and staff have shared in our happy times and supported and encouraged us through the tough times. My husband and I are truly grateful for their excellent veterinary skills and their kindness to us as "parents."

Special acknowledgment is made to Samuel Longer, DVM who founded the clinic in 1964. Many mourn his recent passing. He was a wonderful man who made it a point to get to know not just his patients but their families as well.

Contents

Introduction

People have been sharing their lives with pets for many years. Many a man tells boyhood stories of the dog with whom he shared his bygone childhood. Yet for a long time, those who lived in long term care facilities, rehabilitation centers and psychiatric hospitals were denied the privilege of having pets to interact with and to share their days.

Fortunately, the tide is turning. As the benefits of animal assisted therapy are being recognized, facilities across our nation are implementing pet therapy. Hence the purpose of this guide. Written in simple everyday language, it is designed to assist you in implementing a program no matter how big or small and to be a source of useful information whether you choose to have visiting pets, facility pets or plush animals.

You will find suggestions for starting a program, sample state regulations, facility policies, forms to assist you in staying in compliance with required regulations, questions that you will need to consider before beginning your own program and places to find answers to your questions. Included is a story of pet therapy as it has unfolded at The Masonic Home of New Jersey over the past decade. There is a section devoted to describing what other facilities have done and what changes they would make if they had the chance to do it over again. You will also learn about the resources that are available, types of animals to include and problems that others have experienced.

Most of the information in this book comes from long term care settings, yet it is applicable to any health care setting.

You will not find results of high-tech studies, but rather the stories and results of programs started by people who have tried and, through experience, successfully implemented pet therapy.

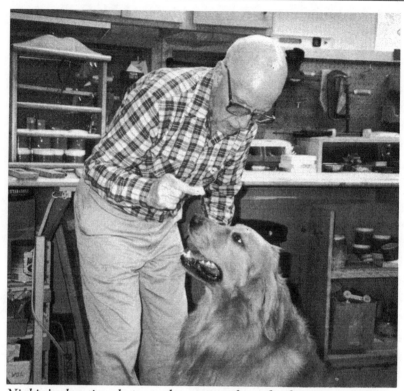

Nickie's day time home, when not making facility visits, is in the woodshop. John Gilbert, our faithful dog walker, takes a break from his woodmaking to give Nickie a treat. Nickie's middle name, John, is in honor of John Gilbert's dedication to our pet therapy program.

Chapter 1

Overview

Why Pet Therapy?

Increasingly, we hear about studies whose results have shown the value of animals in all kinds of therapeutic situations. Reported benefits include reductions in blood pressure and stress levels, shorter recovery periods after illness or surgery and increased capabilities in the areas of safety, self-esteem, spirituality and dealing with loneliness. (Bredenberg, 1990.)

Studies have repeatedly shown that placing live-in pets with the elderly who are institutionalized results in "significant improvements in mood and responsiveness to treatment." (Wallace and Naderman, 1987) Pets can also serve, in the view of many, as a means of "making institutions more humane and less depriving." (Katcher, 1982)

In citing the value of pet therapy programs, Project Life (Jackson, 1990), lists such benefits as inspiring order, routine and opportunities for exercise; promoting socialization, self-esteem, security, conversation and providing affection, entertainment and unqualified acceptance.

Nancy Littell Fox (1979) suggests "A Kitten in a Care Plan" because pets can be a means of providing the tactile stimulation that a person living in a facility often sorely lacks. It is Ms. Fox's contention that there is a special rapport that exists between animals and people.

In a *Time* article, entitled "Furry and Feathery Therapists" (Toufexis, 1987), a study is cited in which it was found that watching fish in an aquarium results in less discomfort for dental surgery patients. Another study mentioned in *Newsweek* was one which showed that the survival rate of patients with serious heart problems was much higher among pet owners (including not only cats and dogs, but chickens, fish and iguanas!) Specific examples of the therapeutic uses of animals, such as a strengthening of motor skills by grooming a rabbit or increasing vocal skills by talking to a cockatiel, were also included in the article.

Those who are disabled or institutionalized often suffer from grief and loneliness. Animals can help in meeting a basic human need by providing unconditional love. Pet therapy can be a wonderful way to enhance the services provided by Activity Professionals. It is hoped that the following articles, personal anecdotes, survey information and sample policies will assist you in implementing the best program for your particular population.

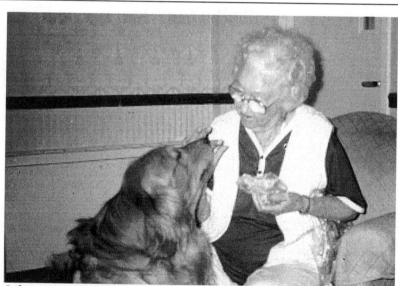

Like many residents, Thelma Tomlinson shares a treat from her "goodie bag" with Nicky.

A Brief History of Pet Therapy

Animals have long played a fascinating and very necessary part in our lives. Over the centuries they have supplied humans with food, clothing, labor and, perhaps most important of all, companionship. Some accounts have even credited pets with giving up their lives in order to save the lives of their masters.

Man and beast have lived together for centuries. In fact, there is archeological evidence to suggest that dogs began to be domesticated as many as 12,000 years ago. Interestingly, it is suggested that this was initiated by the animals themselves, as it freed them from many of the requirements of living in the wild: finding food while competing with other hunters and keeping themselves warm and provided with shelter.

Although the idea of using animals as a therapeutic modality is not a new one and there are many documented cases of their earlier use in restoration and maintenance of health (Bernard, 1988), it was not until the late 1950's that caregivers began to actually recognize the value of some form of animal contact in the daily life of residents in health care settings.

The modern history of pet therapy begins about that time, and, according to Kerry Pechter (1985) can be traced to three landmark events. The first occurred in 1959. A New York child psychiatrist happened to have his pet dog with him when a young, previously unreachable male patient paid him an unexpected visit. The dog licked the face of the boy, who then started smiling and playing with him. Eventually, the boy also warmed up to the doctor, who went on to use pets as ice breakers in his practice and to publish a book in 1969 describing his experiences.

Then, in the mid-1970's, similar results were noted at Ohio State University, where a psychologist kept a kennel of dogs for behavioral studies. Patients in the adjacent psychiatric hospital heard the dogs barking and insisted on seeing them. Visits were arranged, and the trust and affection that resulted between patients and dogs led to the patients' eventual trust of their doctors as well.

The third, and possibly most important, event took place at the University of Pennsylvania in 1980. Researchers interviewing a group of heart attack survivors found that patients *with* pets lived longer after heart attacks than those without and that a relationship existed between pet ownership and lower blood pressure. These three events seemed to support the conclusion that pet ownership helped people to relax and communicate with each other more effectively.

There are literally thousands of wonderful pet stories around the world, many of which could be found to chronicle vital, landmark findings for this history. The author's personal experiences have included witnessing residents who are otherwise non-responsive, reacting to the visit of a warm, friendly animal; observing those who normally never venture from their rooms, walking or otherwise transporting themselves to the first floor lobby areas of our facility to await the arrival of pet visitors; and hearing residents who, though unable to carry on a three minute conversation with humans, can speak to a dog in sensible, structured sentences.

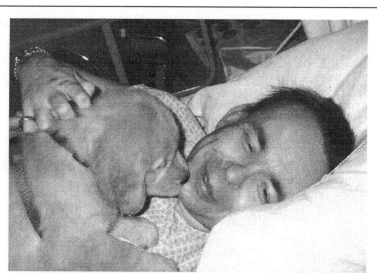

Nicholas John enjoys a visit with Mark Van Houten — or is Mark the one who is enjoying the visit?

The history of pet therapy speaks for itself — its usefulness to humans has been clearly demonstrated. Currently, more and more professionals in health care settings are recognizing a need for people to cohabit with animals and observing that many varieties are well suited to fulfilling this need. States are enforcing laws requiring apartment owners to change their rules and allow residents to own animals.

It only seems natural that people and animals should live together. Or if not live, then at least visit with one another and communicate. Rules and regulations have separated people from animals for a number of years. Fortunately, we are now becoming more aware that animals play a vital role in the well-being of human life, in all its phases and conditions.

Quality of Life Issues and Pet Therapy

As we look to the future of health care, we see that it must be driven by the quality of life issues that surround us. These issues challenge us to provide activities that are more focused on drawing from each resident's own positive life experiences.

While pet therapy is a small part of the pattern of care that we create each day, it may well be one of the most therapeutic interventions we can offer.

An animal's unconditional, unbiased and abiding love is very rewarding to witness in action. It elicits smiles, encourages movement and stimulates conversation, play and interaction. Love from an animal encourages reminiscing, provides nurturing and produces enjoyment. It encourages therapeutic touch, increases self-esteem and, most importantly, provides a home-like atmosphere in any setting.

National surveys show that residents who live in facilities everywhere are concerned about issues like dignity, privacy, staff interactions, facility structure, facility operations and relationships.

Dignity for residents comes from allowing them to make choices for themselves. Their choice to visit with a pet is one that reinforces self-worth and self-esteem as they elaborate about the wonderful pets in their past or the ones they have left with family or friends and even the pets that children or grandchildren now own. Their

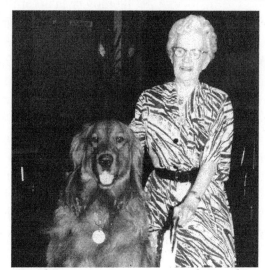

*Carol Bauer enjoys a visit with Bandit as she pushes him around in **her** wheelchair.*

delighted faces and sparkling eyes reflect how they are feeling as they tell their stories. You only have to observe their body language and tone of voice to know that they feel a sense of purpose as they share with others part of who and what they were and continue to be.

Interaction is always a concern when a resident is being introduced to new surroundings or a new group of people. A common denominator, one which can help initiate conversation, may be provided by a pet entering the area. Animals are among the best ice breakers ever invented. Or a staff person may provide this service by mentioning the subject of pets. Whether the resident is a pet lover or not, conversation is quickly initiated.

Dr. Stephen T. Peterson, DVM of International Canine Genetics, Inc. in Malvern, PA wrote to me in a recent correspondence that the "importance of the human-animal bond continues to be recognized for its healing properties." He went on to say that at a recent veterinary conference, *all* the key speakers focused "on the topic of the growing realization of the medical community about the benefits of pet ownership and therapy." So it would seem that we as Activity Professionals should work to provide this very appropriate intervention for the residents that we serve.

We can never begin to know how a program that we institute will touch other lives or exactly what someone may think about its implementation. I was most fortunate to receive the following letter in 1995. It seems to address the areas of the program to which residents, families and pets alike are deeply attached. With regard to the overall benefits of a pet therapy program — I believe the letter on the next page says it all.

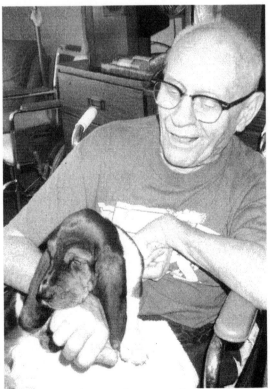

Bud Winters is always ready for some fun. He found this visit with Lady Sadie "B" Good to be a great pleasure.

August 2,1995

Dear Ms. Abdill:

A few weeks ago I received from you a very kind letter and yet another certificate for my contribution to the Pet Therapy program. I am truly sorry that I have never been able to attend one of your Pet Appreciation Night programs. Usually I am away on vacation when they occur. This year I was just back; but, since my new boss did not really approve of my having three weeks off together, I was reluctant to ask right away for another day or afternoon off to come up to New Jersey for the program. Well, maybe next year!

At any rate, I really think some words of appreciation should come to you and the Masonic Home for permitting pets to visit. It means a great deal to me and to Arno. Arno and I are quite close and he does not like to be separated from me for a second. Also, since I come some distance and it takes me four hours to get to the Masonic Home and another four to return, Arno, although he is "only a dog" as people never tire of pointing out to me, is quite a bit of company. And, should I be delayed or forced to stay over due to car trouble or bad weather, I don't have to worry about the dog being home alone, unfed and untended.

But most of all I am so grateful for all the residents and their families whose acquaintance I have made through Arno. On my own, I tend to stick to my own business on the assumption that other people want and are entitled to their own privacy. However, so many people stop me to inquire about what kind of dog Arno is (a Whippet) and may they pet him and what is his name and how old is he, that it frequently takes me twenty minutes to get from the front porch to my mom's room or from her room to my dad's. Arno also has a number of long term "fans" that we have to visit each time as well. I can't tell you how many friendships have started with a resident telling me about a dog he or she once had and misses and then progressing to tell me much more about his or her life and times. At times these secondary trips have really lightened the load a bit when I was feeling down about the condition of my own parents and, at least, made the trip seem worth the effort at times when my own parents have not been very "aware."

So thank you again for the pet therapy program and the progressive philosophy that permits pets to visit the Masonic Home. To me it seems like one of those win-win experiences in that everyone concerned gets something that they need or enjoy.

Yours truly,
John Fragale

Chapter 2

The Masonic Home of New Jersey

Pet Therapy at the Masonic Home

Since the first edition of this manual my facility has grown from 443 to 517 beds. This includes 178 residential beds and 339 medical center beds. During the growth of our facility we have also experienced many changes in our pet therapy program. We are now providing daily pet therapy with two dogs, Prancer and Nicky. We have a full time visitation program — the dogs live with my husband and I and "visit" the facility about forty hours each week. They are both friendly, obedient and crate trained. In fact, a staff member often remarks that he wishes he had been as successful in training his children!

Pet therapy began prior to my arrival as Director of Activities in December 1985. A local animal farm ("Paws" in Mount Laurel, New Jersey) ran a program for schools and nursing facilities and had been making visits to the Masonic Home for several years. They brought four to five animals each time, visited with residents in the solariums, told stories about the animals and allowed the residents to hold, pet and handle them.

Early in 1986 our administrator found an article in a local paper about pet programs in long-term care facilities and suggested that this might be worth looking into. The whole idea greatly interested me so I began gathering articles and information. The more I read, the more I felt that our long-term goal should be to have our own live-in pet and I was definitely leaning toward a dog.

In mid-1986, a staff member suggested, through our Employee Award Program, that plush animals be introduced to the facility. This suggestion was based on an article which said, "Owning and naming a plush animal enhances self-concept, prompts interaction" (Francis and Baly, 1986). So this is how we chose to start. We decided to look for animals that were as close to the real thing as possible, (no pink elephants or green teddy bears!) and the shopping began.

Fortunately, after looking in many stores, we were able to buy animals that met our specifications from an artist in the neighboring town of Willingboro. Carol Cook's artistry and designs were very authentic and she chose fabric that clearly represented the texture of the real animal (e.g. the whale was made of satin and the mallard was made of differently textured wools and blends to show off the feather configuration and give a feathery texture). Some of her creations used in the program included the piglet, mother duck and duckling, sheep, mallard, pony, bunny, whale, mother hen and chicks, lamb and elephant.

We started out by making lists of the residents that we felt could benefit from increased socialization. Carts filled with the plush animals were taken to these residents, who were allowed to choose their own animal. We soon noted that many additional residents were requesting a special "pet" of their own and some wanted more than one. Indeed, we soon found, as suggested, that "Social interest and mental function were significantly higher" (Francis and Baly, 1986) after the implementation of this program.

In 1988, pet policies and procedures were adopted for the facility from state regulations and local township laws. (Copies of the former are included in the *Policies and Procedures* chapter.)

In creating these policies and procedures, the major factors considered were:

- **time:** How much staff time would it take to initiate and carry out the program?
- **cost:** What would be the costs of implementation and upkeep?

- **acceptability:** What would the program's impact be, not only on the Activity Department, but on nursing, housekeeping and all other departments as well?

With these issues in mind, the decision was made to eliminate birds from our initial plans. It was felt that in a facility of our size, with so much family involvement, we might accumulate more birds than could properly be cared for on a daily basis.

After approval of the policy by the Administration and Board, a visiting pet program was formally set up. Fish tanks were also introduced, again at the suggestion of an employee who felt that they would have a soothing effect on some of the residents. The decision was made to purchase six large fish tanks for placement in the medical center solariums.

We initially purchased six thirty-gallon fish tanks with decorative stone and furnishings and six sets of fish. The furnishings included wood stands with front doors, hoods, background paper, gravel, thermometers, air pumps, heaters, filters, drift wood, rocks, shell and plant ornaments. An employee at the store came in, set everything up and provided an in-service training to the staff on care and maintenance. However, please note that the fish tanks did not all live "happily ever after!" They've needed constant attention. Some residents have insisted on feeding the fish bread crusts and other assorted snacks, such as Metamucil. Fish are replaced frequently and one tank was broken by a resident who was agitated. We have also learned that the tanks on our third floor are more difficult to maintain. We attribute this to the warmer temperatures on the higher floors.

We haven't had this problem, but I once heard a noted Activity Professional expounding on the beautiful fish tank she placed in her facility. After a while the fish started to disappear. It took some detective work but they finally discovered that a resident was eating them one by one!

After the fish tanks were in place, the next step was to find a live-in dog. Our veterinarian had strongly recommended a Golden Retriever, so we began searching for one that was suitable. In the meantime, plans for housing the puppy were finalized.

Crate training is a method for house training puppies that substitutes a roomy crate (usually wire or fiberglass) for the den that it would more naturally be raised in. It seemed to be the method of choice; those who had used them claimed that crates were a wonderful invention. Initially, many pet owners have a negative reaction, feeling that crates are cages and certainly shouldn't be a part of the way they want to treat their new, loving puppy. But Nicki Meyer (1984) suggests that crates facilitate good feelings for puppies, who see the world differently from us. A young puppy instinctively seeks the comfort and safety of a den and since he does not want to soil his living area, he will become housebroken more quickly. (This article is included in the chapter on dogs.) It has also been my own personal experience that crates are helpful in providing dogs with a place to call their own. Over the years I have concluded that every dog deserves a crate. Not just for the puppy stage but for all of its life.

Word soon got out that a puppy was about to take up residence at the Home. The daughter-in-law of Ottilie Powell, one of our residents, had often brought her Siberian Huskies to visit through the visiting pet program and had heard about our search for a puppy. She offered to donate one of her puppies to us. They were beautiful animals and very well behaved, so we decided to take her up on the offer. We were given the opportunity to choose between two beautiful male pups who were brought to the home and "King," the one with the matching powder blue eyes, was selected. He was a charmer; those blue eyes would dazzle anyone. He would surely become the perfect pet.

A large crate was purchased and the Maintenance Department installed slats. They made the crate small to begin with, but allowed for possible enlargement as the puppy grew.

The dog's shots were current, but a health certificate was needed, so off to the veterinarian we went. On July 8, 1988 schedules were made and the program was in full swing.

Initially, nine residents wanted to take part in the dog's care. However, within two weeks, only two of the original nine were able to fulfill their responsibilities and a new schedule was formulated. The Activity Staff cared for him from 8:00 a.m. to 4:00 p.m. and the two residents cared for him during the evening hours. Backup care was provided by the nursing and security departments.

A local trainer evaluated him and deemed him to be a suitable candidate, so dominance/obedience training began. By October of 1988, King had completed puppy training and in August 1989, he received his obedience course degree in the Subnovice class.

Everyone loved King. When he was not on the floors with an Activity Assistant, he stayed in the Activity Room on a leash, though it soon became obvious that the leash was not his choice. He kissed and played happily with visitors, but howled when they left. He would hold onto their hands or arms to encourage them to stay; this of course, was not acceptable. He also became more and more resistant to returning to the crate after his evening walk.

One of the nurses offered to take him home and bring him back with her each day. This seemed to be a good solution since she had a fenced-in yard in which he could run. But in mid-May, she reported that King had killed a neighbor's rabbit, was guarding it and no one could get near him. Since the rabbit had not been mauled or dismembered in any way, it was decided that it had probably died of fright when King made an attempt to play with it. Apparently King himself was afraid and felt that he was protecting the rabbit, but this was more than our nurse had bargained for.

So King went home with me that night. Since we knew he would not get along with the dog we already had, they were kept in separate quarters and King went to work with me every day.

By mid-summer, King's undesirable traits had grown worse: he howled when left on his leash, would not obey commands and grabbed residents' arms or hands in an attempt to prevent them from leaving after a visit. This was not a problem for staff but was for residents, many of whom had delicate skin. The decision was made to remove King from the facility and since my husband and I had grown attached to him, we adopted him as a family pet, a role for which he was admirably suited.

The search then began for a replacement. This time we decided to follow the veterinarian's advice and look for a Golden Retriever. A well-respected breeder in the area was expecting a litter to be born around Christmas 1990 and promised to let us know when they arrived. However, in August she called and said that another breeder, with whom she bred her dogs, had a handsome puppy who had been returned to him. The owner, an older gentleman, had fallen ill and could no longer care for this frisky six month old.

Our new therapy dog was already named "Bandit" and what an appropriate name it turned out to be! Since he needed instruction before beginning his new job, we traveled four hours every weekend for Bandit's obedience training.

It was not long before we realized who it was that was being trained! The instructor and my husband would look on while I worked Bandit in the large back yard. On two occasions Bandit had not mastered his last week's lesson well enough, so he had to repeat them until he did. I nearly gave up when it came to the "down" command, but we were finally able to accomplish it and move on.

One important lesson I learned was that dogs require a lot of praise. After observing me rewarding Bandit with a hug and kiss, the trainer said "Don't love him up — praise him!" And this we continued to do. It was an enjoyable time — watching Bandit grow and learn to respond to verbal commands.

During those six months of training, I would occasionally take Bandit to the facility in the evening hours. Gradually he was introduced to the slippery floors, the strange noises in the stair wells, the sounds of the elevator doors opening and closing and all those chairs with the big wheels. He learned quickly. I was amazed one night at the way he sniffed his way to my husband's office (he also works at the Home) without a clue from me. Bandit was a smart dog and he was winning the hearts of residents and staff alike.

As he visited more frequently, he soon learned his boundaries and was able to roam freely within the Activity Room. He visited with residents who came every day to do crafts, as well as with the not-so-frequent visitors. Many of those coming from outside the facility were amazed to see that a dog was part of the Activity Department.

For many months Bandit visited regularly with the residents in the medical center and played games with one of our groups of residents who were severely cognitively impaired. He would gently fetch a large foam ball from each resident and return it to the handler, who remained in the center of the horseshoe. He was a wonderful addition to our pet therapy program. Often sitting in the chair just inside my office door, he would extend his paw to anyone who crossed the threshold.

Just one more step remained…Bandit was not an official "Therapy Dog." So I set out to find an evaluator who would do the necessary testing. On February 15, 1992 Bandit tested and qualified for his Canine Good Citizen Certificate and completed his requirements for "Therapy Dog" certification through Therapy Dogs International.

However, the story does not end there. Bandit had passed the test, yet he became more and more aggressive. He was living up to his name and I never knew what he would steal next. He could sniff out a cookie or cracker from a wheelchair bag and nose dive in to retrieve it before I knew what was happening. Residents were losing candy and tissues. Although no one seemed to mind, I knew this was not acceptable. One day during a session in the Medical Center, Bandit had stolen a linen hankie — and made it disappear — like magic. He also become overbearing in my office. He wanted to be in the middle of everything. His attention-getting antics became more than I could handle. I knew this behavior could not continue and that he could not remain in the facility. It happened that as I came to this conclusion, two gentleman were sitting in a hallway. After a brief visit with Bandit, as I was walking away, one said to the other "Isn't this a wonderful place?" And the other replied, "Yes it is and now it's a real home. We have our own dog!"

I knew the program could not be lost. I also knew from my research that there were plenty of very successful therapy dog programs around. By accepting a beautiful Huskie as our first dog we'd disregarded the advice we'd been given about breeds; the second time we'd taken in a dog who had already developed bad habits. There had to be a dog that would work out. After some consultation with the vets and the breeders, we decided to purchase a new puppy. I made arrangements to purchase a puppy from a litter that would be ready to leave home on June 12, 1992. I left the selection up to the breeder, making it very clear that this puppy *must* work out.

When the puppies were about five weeks old, we went with friends to see the litter and to hold the precious pup that we hoped would soon become the perfect therapy pet for our program. The breeder walked out of her house with Moses. He did turn out to be the perfect pet. His personality was ideal. The residents loved him and cared for him during the day. He was intelligent, he learned quickly, he was everything we could have ever wanted. Yet, again our program would be disrupted, this time by Moses' untimely death. Little did we know at the time of the deadly circumstances that could arise from the use of choke chains. On the Saturday before Thanksgiving 1992, while he was playing with Bandit in the yard, Moses became the victim of a choke chain accident. It was a most unhappy time. We had to plan how we would inform the residents. It was a sad day in our facility as the news traveled. I personally made rounds to inform the residents directly involved in his care. Many tears were shed. Residents and staff along with volunteers and visitors shared the sorrow of Moses' death. Announcements were created for the bulletin boards. An "In Memoriam" was placed in the next issue of the "Home Team," a facility newspaper.

In the midst of all this sadness I knew that this was a program that must continue.

Bandit was brought back to the facility. My thinking was that perhaps being almost a year older he would be more settled. But he was more active than ever.

It soon become apparent that the solution was to find a new puppy. Even though I knew there could never be another Moses, there *had* to be another puppy to fit the bill. We were most fortunate in hearing of a new litter that would be ready for homes on December 20, 1992. But, we pondered, was it too fast to bring in a new puppy? Should we wait three to six months for the healing process to occur? A decision had to be made quickly if we were to purchase a puppy from this new litter. The final decision was to get a new puppy as soon as possible. The Pentals, of Golden Haven Golden Retrievers in Denton, Maryland, assured me that we would indeed be able to have it on December 20th. I could not think of a better way to fill the void that Moses' absence had created, especially with the holidays so quickly approaching. What better way to brighten the lives of our many residents than to have a visit from a new Golden Retriever puppy on Christmas morning?

And so it was that year that our traditional Christmas morning visits from Santa included not only a visit from the jolly old man himself and a Christmas stocking filled with goodies, but Christmas morning, 1992 would also be a morning of sharing new life, new hope and much happiness. Nicholas John Firman of the Woodshop ("Nicky" as he became known) was carried throughout the facility in a basket. Watching the reactions of our residents gave me one of the most rewarding Christmas mornings I have spent at the Home. There were twinkling eyes, arms reaching out, hugs, kisses and cuddles and even a tear glistened as residents marveled over this adorable new puppy that would become a wonderful part of our Masonic Home family.

Nicky grew not only in size to his current ninety pounds— he grew into a perfect therapy dog. He seems to sense the fragility of our residents and is gentle with them, yet he also knows he can play ball and fetch with the folks that are more active. And he knows he can be a dog at home with his brothers. Playing together and being just a good old dog.

But the program has been even further enhanced with the addition of Prancer in January 1993. Little did my husband and I ever expect to have four dogs! Nor, when we agreed to take Prancer, did we expect to have another therapy dog. Our friend, Ron Howard, who was the breeder and trainer for Bandit, had passed away just a few short months after cancer surgery. His wife, Lynn, was looking for homes for the dogs and we agreed to take a male. Lynn said that Prancer would make a wonderful therapy dog and he did. He quickly adapted to his new home. I had thought that he would need a slow introduction to the facility since it was so big, had slippery floors and so many new things, such as paging, to which he would have to become accustomed.

To my delight and surprise, he was a natural. What was to be a two-to-three hour session on a Saturday morning ended up being a six hour session that ended with Prancer in the Medical Center — off the leash — visiting from room to room, sitting beside chairs and delighting residents with whom he stopped to visit.

This was a dream come true day for me. Now I had two dogs who would work in our program.

So our van was housed with two crates in the back. Now each day Nicky and Prancer leave for work with us while King and Bandit hang out together at home. Two therapy dogs, yet two very different personalities. While Nicky has more of a happy-go-lucky personality, Prancer is more laid back. Nicky spends his day in the Woodshop with his handler Pat Mitchell, where many residents visit him on a daily basis. She also takes him to the Medical Center for one-on-one visits. Prancer on the other hand, spends the day with me. He follows me wherever I go, making stops along the way for some affectionate hugs and petting. When I'm busy in my office, he sleeps or sits on a chair next to my secretary's desk. He extends his paw to those who come to pet him and give him hugs. If he is sleeping in my office the residents know to just call him and tell him "Up" and he perches on the chair to share some time together with them.

For now my program is in place and working well. Yet there is so much room for growth. Available time is the only thing holding me back. Some day our program may grow to include a cat, perhaps a rabbit and who knows what else? In the mean time, Nicky and Prancer are providing the unconditional love and all the other benefits a pet therapy program can provide.

Pet Therapy For Alzheimer's: Does It Really Work?

It has been my experience that, yes, Pet Therapy does in fact work, but only under the direct supervision of a handler. Just the entrance of one of our dogs on the special care unit seems to brighten the spirits of most residents, not to mention the reaction that it gets from the staff. Staff members from every discipline want to visit with the dog. Whether they share a handshake or a hug, everyone seems happier for the experience.

For those on the unit who are still ambulatory, walking a dog can be most therapeutic: stimulating conversation and reminiscences and producing joy over the ability to spend time with an animal. It has been my experience that the residents do not recognize the dog in the present, rather they elaborate on the dog they remember. Example: One of our residents speaks constantly about how our dog kisses her and sits on her lap whenever she sits down. However, the dog that she actually walks on the unit *never* has kissed her. He just does not kiss anyone, he weighs 75 pounds and is *not* a "lap dog." This type of conversation, however, can lead to the gathering of pertinent information about a resident.

The most serious problem that can face an animal in such a setting might arise if a resident lashes out verbally or physically and scares the animal. This type of behavior towards an animal could *possibly* cause the animal to exhibit "fear aggression" or could instill fear in an animal. If the animal exhibits "fear aggression," it may growl, snarl and show its teeth or even bite the resident engaged in the lashing out behavior. If the animal is frightened, it may remember the experience and not want to enter that particular area of the facility on its next rounds. If an incident such as lashing out occurs, the animal may exhibit new behavior as a reaction to it. If no one witnesses the episode, however, you will never know the cause of this new behavior. For this reason, I believe that an animal should *always* be accompanied by a handler when in the presence of residents with Alzheimer's or dementia-type diseases.

Another interesting observation regarding residents who are cognitively impaired is that residents can remember our dogs names, yet can't begin to tell you the names of our staff. We have also recognized that they remember the pet handler in our facility as "the dog lady," yet they do not recall her name. We also found that one resident, who as a rule never spoke in complete or comprehensible sentences, could tell us a complete story about her dog from her childhood days. This assisted us in obtaining valuable information about her past. In summary, pet therapy does work with residents who have Alzheimer's by stimulating increased socialization, memory recall and movement, as well as providing therapeutic touch and a general sense of well being.

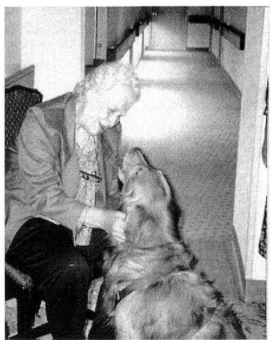

Cynthia Lepore is thrilled by a visit from Nicky. She says, "He is just beautiful." and loves his friendly disposition.

Pet Therapy: Some Unexpected Perks

Pet therapy, like any other adventure, can bring the unexpected into your life.

Besides the fact that pet therapy brings obvious benefits to its providers in general, it has brought two exceptional experiences to my own life:

The first experience occurred in March of 1989. Our group of Therapy Dogs International volunteers had made contact with a local television program, AM Philadelphia. The TV station agreed to come to our facility to tape their March visit. On April 4, 1989 the show was aired. We were very excited to have TV coverage of such a valuable program. Not only were the Therapy Dogs International dogs and the handlers interviewed, but they also included "King" — our then aspiring facility pet and interviewed us in regards to the reasons for implementing such a program.

In the second case, a friend of mine was writing a romance novel. It was a story about an Activity Director — she hit a snag in writing the book and suddenly realized that an energetic Golden Retriever would provide the added spark that the book needed. The book was published with a dedication that read:

> *This book is dedicated to the thousands of Activity Professionals across the nation who provide service to the elderly, the infirm and the handicapped, tirelessly giving so much of themselves in performing this valuable work.*
>
> *Special thanks to Margaret Abdill, Director of Activities at the Masonic Home of New Jersey, whose knowledge of the profession was of such great help in preparing this book, and to Bandit, Therapy Dog at the MHNJ, the inspiration for Sunny.*

I was privileged to travel with the author, Beverly Haaf, to civic organizations and to four book signings with Bandit. I was also able to enlighten people who came to these events about the field of activity programming, pet therapy and advancements in long-term care.

Sometimes it was amusing. While at one of our book signings, a lady was asking me about Bandit and why he was allowed in the mall. I explained that he was a Therapy Dog and had been at the Home since he was about one year old. She looked at me with a questioning face and said, "Oh, what's wrong with him that he needs a nursing home?" As she finished her question her face became bright red and she said, "I'm out of here" and left.

A year after the book was published, the New Jersey Activity Professionals used the theme "Activities: The Best Seller" for their annual convention. Beverly was our keynote speaker and the book was one of the "freebies" included in our registration bags. We again had a book signing where Bandit was present to share in the festivities.

I have also had the opportunity to write articles for the Masonic Newspaper in New Jersey, featuring our Pet Therapy program.

The list of perks that can occur is endless, I'm sure. But the best perk of all is seeing the faces of my residents when one of the dogs pays a visit.

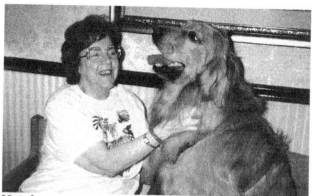

Doris Heinlein enjoys a friendly visit from Nickie as he makes his rounds through the home. Residents like Doris love to run their hands through his warm, thick fur.

Chapter 3

Program Implementation

Research and development are a necessary part of creating a new program. Pet therapy programs are no exception to this rule. The suggestions that follow will provide information on some of the issues that need to be considered.

Where Do I Begin?

Before starting, the following questions need to be considered:

- Is this program feasible for me and my facility/agency?
- Is time available for development and implementation?
- Will the costs be reasonable and compatible with budgetary constraints?
- What does the facility's governing body think of pet programs?
- Can other disciplines be counted on to cooperate? (It is usually a good idea to have an interdisciplinary meeting to determine this and to gain support and input.)
- Can our staff handle this new obligation?
- Who will be the main person responsible for the care and health of the pet(s); for purchase and quality control after the program's implementation?
- Who will provide back-up support?
- What roles can residents or clients play?
- If housing a pet in the facility 24 hours a day, who will care for it when the Activity Staff is not there?
- Who will handle emergencies if the Activity Staff is not available?
- Which veterinarian will provide health care for the pet?

Perhaps one of the most important cautions to keep in mind is that if you are planning to establish a facility pet, *you* are the one responsible for its care after its arrival. For example, Mrs. Smith's granddaughter may be an expert when it comes to breeding and raising expensive, exotic birds and is happy to donate one to your facility, However, you will need to keep it alive and well once it has been placed in your care. Are you prepared to provide the time and money demanded to keep such a delicate animal alive?

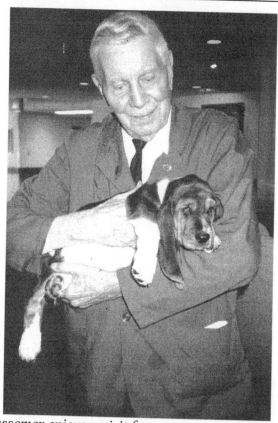

Anton Hassemer enjoys a visit from a new puppy, Lady Sadie "B" Good

You will need information about applicable city or township regulations, as well as animal licensing regulations. The regulations and requirements of the state agency that controls pets in facilities must also be determined. More importantly, you must decide if they can be met.

It might be helpful to contact other Activity Professionals in your area through local and state organizations, to learn what their experiences have been in implementing such a program.

Administrative support for your program is absolutely essential. However, before enlisting this support try to make some decisions about the species of animal and the type of program which could be implemented. Have your facts straight when first presenting this information and include the projected initial and on-going benefits and costs. It might be helpful to also include some documentation of the state or federal government's position, the results gained elsewhere with programs of this type and some brief suggestions for policies and procedures.

Types Of Pet Therapy

1. **Facility pets/full time residency**
   a) Animals that live in the facility twenty-four hours a day — for example, dogs, cats, rabbits, fish, birds, mice, rats or guinea pigs
2. **Facility pets/full time visitation** (New Jersey regulations — four or more hours a day)
   a) Provided by staff members willing to bring their pets in on a regularly scheduled basis
   b) Provided by a facility-owned pet that is cared for by a full-time staff member and brought in daily
3. **Periodic pet visitations/**
   a) Pets from organized groups:
      1) Local training clubs

    2) Groups of therapy dogs who have passed special training programs and are deemed worthy of the certification to visit in special-need settings

    3) Local animal/humane societies or shelters

    4) 4-H Clubs

  b) Families or visitors

    1) Programs in which families or visitors bring in their own pets

    2) Programs in which families or visitors bring in the resident's own personal pets

4. **Animal contacts — outside trips**

  a) Local zoos

  b) Area animal farms or habitats (Check with local elementary schools for such agencies.)

5. **Animal contacts — natural surroundings**

  a) Don't forget about birds living in the wild; they need to be fed in the winter. This can be accomplished by simply installing feeders and buying bird seed. Caution: someone must keep feeders filled, as birds come to depend on them.

  b) In areas where deer or small animals might be sighted, encourage the residents to look out their windows and view the scenery. A contest could be developed around spotting the greatest variety of animals in a month, especially in a rural area where groundhogs and raccoons come out in early evening and deer can be seen along the edge of the woods.

6. **Plush animals**

Even if you program can't accommodate live animals, you can still use plush animals and gain many of the same benefits.

Also see the next chapter on *Activities* for ideas on the ways you can use pets as part of your activity program.

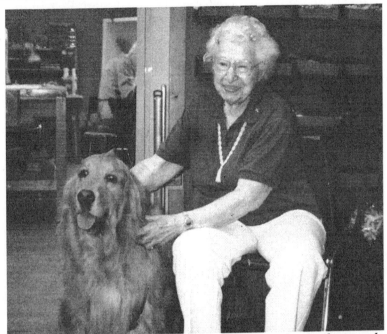

Anna Votapek visits with Nickie almost every day in the wood shop. Normally Nickie rolls over on his back so Anna can rub his belly. Today they chose a more formal pose.

Choosing The Right Pet For You

The first rule in choosing a pet is to remember that it is more important to find the *right* animal than to find *an* animal. Think about how much time and money could be wasted if the animal you have purchased is the wrong choice. (This can easily happen, as this author can attest from personal experience!) Choose carefully and you will spare residents the grief that removal of a pet from the facility might bring. But if a mistake *is* made, remember that we are all only human. Experience is never wasted; just consider how much more you will know the second time around!

Direct contact with a breeder can be very useful. Be honest with the breeder. If you are not an expert on selecting the right pet, tell them what you are looking for and have them select the best choice for you from the litter. A good breeder should be able to assist in temperament-testing the animal chosen or suggest someone who can. (*Note*: Never take a puppy who leaves the pack to check you out. Choose one that is laid back, a "wimpy" one.) Trainers in your area may also be helpful. They might be able to put you in touch with people who have older, trained show animals. Some of these animals often fail in competition or retire early for various reasons, but still make excellent therapy pets.

If you have selected fish, look into the possibility of a local store setting up the tanks. Look for a store that has a good reputation and is not likely to overcharge or sell inferior equipment. Inquire if there is an advisor or staff person who will assist you when problems arise. The store from which our tanks were purchased advised that we not begin with the usual "starter tanks." These are designed for people who are not sure what they really want. They enable them to embark on a new adventure without spending large sums of money. Facility budgets do not often allow for the replacement of equipment, so no matter what your choice, it is better to start with good quality equipment.

Constantly assess all areas of the program, including the appropriateness of the animals selected. Make necessary changes in the program to meet the changing needs of those it serves.

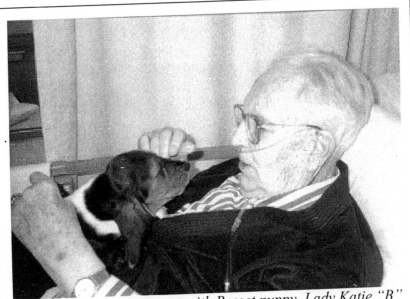

Lester Ely enjoys a moment with Basset puppy, Lady Katie "B" Good.

Staff Responsibilities

The best way to handle this matter is to draw up a plan that specifies all duties, who will perform them, when they will be done and who the back-up will be. Determine if the pet can be cared for most properly if it lives within the facility 24 hours a day or if it can be cared for at home and only brought in during working hours. Be prepared — if your facility has three hundred residents and three hundred employees, that's how many opinions you will get on "how to do things the right way." So have your plan on paper, well defined and ready to implement when your choice of animal arrives. Be sure your plan specifies the following: who will feed the animal and when; who will take care of housekeeping for the areas the animal will occupy; where and when the animal will be walked and who will do it; when and where the pet will nap.

Some pets sleep 70% of the day. They need a place to nap after an hour of work.

Gain support from other department heads who can inform their staff about proper procedures to follow for your new addition. Hold a brainstorming session and try to determine ways of handling any difficult situations that might arise. Draw up some simple guidelines so residents and visitors will know the rules. (An important point to stress is exactly *who is and who is not* allowed to feed the animals.)

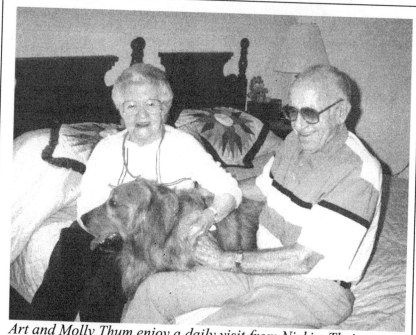

Art and Molly Thum enjoy a daily visit from Nickie. Their room is just down the hall from the woodshop. He knows his way to their room where he usually gets a special treat and a lot of hugs.

Some suggestions if you decide to set up a visitation program and wish to allow visitors to bring in their pets:

- Place a poster in the reception area to inform visitors about the program.
- Include this information in any manual or handbook that you will be giving out to new residents or families:
  - types of pets allowed in your facility.
  - details about how an animal is to be registered and where this registration is to be handled.
  - ground rules for the pet visitor: clearly state that it must be well-groomed, controlled by leash or verbal command, up-to-date on shots, be licensed in its town/city/borough of residence, be signed in and out of the Pet Registration book and most important of all, be well mannered and *not* show signs of aggressive behavior.

Veterinary Care

This is one of the most important decisions that you can make in the planning stage of your program. It is essential that you not wait until your pet arrives to select the veterinarian or veterinary group that will care for your pet. Tell the veterinarian(s) about your intent to set up a pet therapy program. Let them know where your facility is located and who besides yourself might be calling or bringing the pet in for checkups or emergency care. Be sure they know how your billing office prefers to handle bills and be sure they are willing to work with you. They will probably be able to provide helpful information about local breeders, routine care, approximate costs and the development of policies and procedures. Also ask their opinion about local trainers and special training for your pet. (Don't be afraid to ask questions; you will in effect be getting your information "straight from the horse's mouth.")

Remember, if this pet is your first, you may find yourself spending a lot of time at the vet's or on the phone. After our first facility dog (King) arrived, I picked the vets' brains for months. Dr. Longer, Dr. Wolf and Dr. Kimmelman were more than kind to me and never seemed annoyed by my many questions and frequent visits.

I can't say enough about the doctors who have worked in the clinic we chose. Each one has been there to provide excellent care for new puppies, sick dogs or routine checkups. There is sure to be a veterinary practice like this in your area. Check around and find it! The peace of mind that comes from knowing you have good veterinary care is only a phone call away.

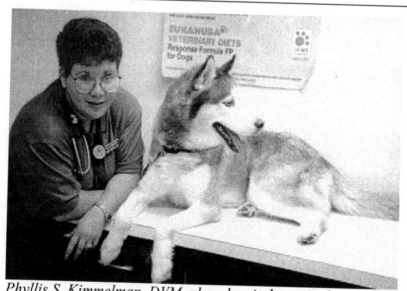

Phyllis S. Kimmelman, DVM, played a vital part in the early stages of my pet therapy program. King made many visits to the clinic and I always had a list of questions for her.

Chapter 4

Activities

This chapter looks at some of the activities you can do with pets. As you will see, a creative pet therapy program can make use of many different kinds of animals (including plush animals) and take place in many different locations.

Pets may be used to meet the needs of residents at many different levels of cognitive, physical and emotional functioning. If we look at the eight levels of resident functioning described by Elizabeth Best Martini (1997), we see that pets can provide activities for each of the first seven levels.

Level 1: Sensory Integration. Animals are a sensory integration experience all by themselves providing sight and sound, smell and feeling experiences all linked together in one animal.

Level 2: Sensory Stimulation. Each of the separate aspects of an animal stimulates the senses. Holding and petting an animal is especially effective.

Level 3: Validation. This is for people who are still able to communicate but are not oriented to person, place and/or time. Validation is accomplished by listening to the experiences that the resident or client talks about. It doesn't matter if they are accurate. You are validating the person's worth by listening.

Level 4: Remotivating and Reminiscing. This is one of he easiest levels. Many people just seem to talk more and care more about life when animals are around.

Level 5: Resocializing. Animals are an automatic center for a group to form around. In resocializing, the group meets to come up with appropriate ways to take care of the pets as members of a community.

Level 6: Cognitive Stimulation and Retraining. This can be accomplished more easily with a good motivator. The chance to work with animals is often an appropriate motivation.

Level 7: Short Term Rehab. This level of care tends to focus more on medical issues, but visits from pets can provide a useful and appropriate change of pace. A hectic therapy schedule, especially when you fatigue easily or hurt, causes stress. Interacting with animals has been shown to reduce stress levels in many situations.

Level 8: Community Integration. This level of care is usually focused on relearning skills in the community outside of the facility, but much of the motivation for getting back into the community can come from wanting to take care of facility pets.

This experience may also lead the resident to ask for a therapy dog to help out once they are at home. Therapy dogs can be specially trained as leader guide dogs, or as dogs which will pick up items or signal that the phone is ringing.

As you look through this chapter (and the rest of the book) remember that these are only a few of the possible activities you can do with animals. Be creative and look for ways that the natural bond between animals and people can bring out the best in both.

1. Animal Visits Throughout The Facility

Group Size: Individual room visits or small groups gathered in common areas

Time: One hour (Note: One hour indicates the time the animal will be in the facility — not each individual unit)

Formation: None

Materials: Pets' bowls for water breaks, paper towels and trash bags to clean up any accidents, camera (optional) to capture faces of the residents for posters for the facility or publicity for local newspapers and/or brochures, towelettes for residents to wash hands after handling the pets. (Soap and water hand washing is preferable to just using towelettes. Have residents wash their hands *before* touching the animals to reduce the amount of germs placed on the animal's coat.)

Benefits

Physical: uses eye-hand coordination, exercises prehension actions, encourages active range of motion, supports kinesthetic awareness of body parts and physical actions, exercises a variety of sensory neurons including smell, touch and pressure awareness, encourages both lateral and bilateral movements, allows use of spatial awareness in relationship to other objects.

Mental: encourages use of past knowledge (labeling, naming, describing), exercises use of short term and long term memory, invites use of concentration skills (alternatives, focusing and selecting; intermittent or continuous intensity of concentration; brief, average and long duration of attention), encourages use of both receptive and expressive communication skills.

Emotional: increases options for emotional release of stress, allows sense of belonging, offers opportunities to express feelings, stimulates memory of past feelings.

Spiritual: encourages compassion and caring; calls for
gentleness, kindness and self-control; invites the resident to
be present in the "here and now."

Social: encourages social interactions with others patterns
include little/average/much and intermittent/continuous;
uses a variety of social style interactions including
cooperative, parallel, sharing and stewardship; offers
opportunities for communication and cohort support.

Greetings

- Knock at each door if not open and ask if you may enter
  with a visitor and a pet. Do not proceed with visit if
  resident shows fear of animals, has conflicting health
  diagnoses or does not wish to participate.
- Introduce yourself as well as the pet and pet handler if
  unknown to the resident.
- If visiting a common area (e.g., solarium or sun porch) ask
  if you may come in and visit with the handler and the pet.
  Do not proceed with common area visits if anyone shows
  fear of the pet, has conflicting health diagnoses or does not
  wish to participate. If the residents not desiring to
  participate express their willingness to leave the common
  area, thank them and offer assistance, then proceed with the
  visit.
- Lead off the conversation with questions such as, "Did you
  ever have a pet?" and "What kind was it?"

Activity

Facility-wide animal-assisted activities can be accomplished
with a variety of animals (dogs, cats, birds, pigs, rabbits or
virtually any animal your state or facility allows in your
program). Preplanning needs to begin by scheduling the visit
on the monthly calendar. Additional reminders should follow
your facility's usual procedure (posters on bulletin boards,
screens for community bulletin boards on TV system, flyers to
residents' rooms and/or verbal reminders by staff). Staff and/or

volunteers need to be scheduled to escort the handlers through the facility, unless they are regular visitors familiar with your policies and procedures. The pets will be taken either to residents' rooms or common areas. Remember that they need to be under control with a leash and/or verbal command or carried in a basket, box or small crate. Small animals should never be carried next to your body to avoid overheating. Use either a residential pet or schedule 1-6 handlers depending on the size of your facility. It is best to schedule more than one pet since handlers sometimes must cancel due to their own personal conflicts or a problem with the animal.

Discussion Starters
- Did you ever see a pet like this ?
- Do you know what it is (i.e. specific breed)?
- How many pets did you have?
- Do you know how much time it takes to care for a pet like this?
- Does your family have any pets?
- Do any of your family or friends bring pets to visit you?
- If you could have a pet now, what kind would you like to have?

2. Plush Animal Activity

Group Size: 1:1 visits
Time: 5 to 10 minutes
Formation: Sit by the bedside of the resident or sit by the chair they are sitting in so as to be at eye level.
Materials: Each resident's plush animal.

Benefits

Physical: uses eye-hand coordination, exercises prehension actions, encourages active range of motion, supports kinesthetic awareness of body parts and physical actions, exercises a variety of sensory neurons including visual perception differences in surface texture, color and variations in size and shape, touch (weave, composition, material, structure coarseness) and pressure awareness, encourages both lateral and bilateral movements, allows use of spatial awareness in relationship to other objects.

Mental: encourages use of past knowledge (labeling, naming, describing, recalling), exercises use of short term and long term memory, invites use of concentration skills (alternatives, focusing and selecting; intermittent or continuous intensity of concentration; brief, average and long duration of attention), encourages use of both receptive and expressive communication skills.

Emotional: increases options for emotional release of stress, allows sense of belonging, offers opportunities to express feelings, stimulates memory of past feelings, allows for emotional expression and satisfaction through hugging and caressing plush animal.

Spiritual: encourages compassion and caring; calls for gentleness, kindness and self-control; invites the resident to be present in the "here and now."

Social: encourages social interactions with others (patterns including little/average/much, intermittent/continuous);

uses a variety of social style interactions including cooperative, parallel, sharing and stewardship; offers opportunities for communication.

Greetings
- Stop by the resident's room and make eye contact.
- Introduce yourself if unknown to the resident.
- Ask if you might come in and visit for a while.

Activity
This activity is a one-to-one visit to enhance the therapeutic value of a plush animal for the resident. It's a good idea to provide introductory information that is available to all staff to assist them in knowing the value of pet therapy and how to enhance the program through visits and conversation.

Conversation Starters
- Ask the resident how s/he obtained his/her plush animal.
- Ask the name of the animal.
- Ask why the animal is special.
- Ask if s/he had a real animal like the plush one earlier in his/her lifetime.
- Ask if you might touch the animal and hold it for a moment.
- Give the animal a hug and tell the person how much you like it, too.
- Inquire if you might come again to visit.
- Conclude the visit by asking if you might give the person a hug.

3. Dog Training School Demo

Group Size: 40 to 100 people
Time: One hour
Formation: In an auditorium or a large room, place residents in long rows on either side facing the center of the room. Do not block doorways.
Materials: Mats and equipment supplied by training school, pin-on microphone to allow instructor or handler to work independently of hand-held microphones and dangerous wires.

Benefits

Physical: provides opportunity to demonstrate static and sitting balance through the use of accurate and prompt postural adjustments to body movements to maintain balance; encourages use of good placement of body weight appropriately placed over buttocks with the torso and head held in vertical alignment over the hips.

Mental: encourages use of attention span including attention to task, motor quietness, cognitive focus and the ability to ignore interruptions and impulsive thoughts; encourages use of past knowledge (labeling, naming, describing); exercises use of short term and long term memory, invites use of concentration skills (alternatives, focusing and selecting; intermittent or continuous intensity of concentration; brief, average and long duration of attention).

Emotional: increases options for emotional release of stress, allows sense of belonging, stimulates memory of past feelings, provides opportunities to obtain knowledge to share with others (e.g., visiting family members) allowing pride in one's knowledge.

Spiritual: invites the resident to be present in the "here and now;" allows one to "journey with" others through shared knowledge and experiences.

Social: allows the practice of appropriate social skills related to audience behaviors; provides opportunities to obtain information to share with others at a future date.

Activity

Have the residents sitting in positions where they can see the center of the room where the dogs will be performing.

Conversation Starters

- Ask the owner or instructor to give some background information about the school.
- Ask the handlers or instructors to tell:
  - the commands and the performance accuracy of each command.
  - the name, the breed and the age of each dog.
  - how long it takes a dog to get to the performance level at which they are working.

4. Animal Farm/Shelter/Zoo Visits

Group Size: 10 to 20 people
Time: One hour
Formation: Horseshoe
Materials: The animals, lap covers, towelettes, paper towels, trash
bags, disposable water bowls. (Soap and water hand washing is
preferable to just using towelettes. Have residents wash their
hands *before* touching the animals to reduce the amount of
germs placed on the animals' coats.)

Benefits

Physical: uses eye-hand coordination; exercises prehension
actions; encourages active range of motion; supports
kinesthetic awareness of body parts and physical actions;
exercises a variety of sensory neurons including smell,
touch and pressure awareness; allows use of spatial
awareness in relationship to other objects.

Mental: encourages use of past knowledge (labeling, naming,
describing); exercises use of short term and long term
memory; invites use of concentration skills (alternatives,
focusing and selecting; intermittent or continuous intensity
of concentration; varied durations of attention), encourages
use of both receptive and expressive communication skills

Emotional: increases options for emotional release of stress,
allows sense of belonging, offers opportunities to express
feelings, stimulates memory of past feelings.

Spiritual: encourages compassion and caring; calls for
gentleness, kindness and self-control; invites the resident to
be present in the "here and now."

Social: encourages varied social interactions with others; uses a
variety of social style interactions including cooperative,
parallel, sharing and stewardship; offers opportunities for
communication and cohort support; provides opportunities
to obtain information to share with others at a future date.

Greetings

Welcome the group and describe the organization that is providing the activity. Briefly tell participants where the visitors are located, explain their funding and how many animals they house. Introduce the handlers to the group. Variations to this include introducing the residents individually or to asking the residents to introduce themselves.

Activity

Provide a cart to transport crates from the entrance to the location of the activity. Have the residents sit in a horseshoe so that the handlers may easily pick up the animals from their crates and proceed from resident to resident with each individual animal. Introduce the handlers and explain what type of agency they come from. Arrange for staff and volunteers to assist the handlers, if appropriate, to take the animals to each resident to hold, touch or stroke. Be sure the room is well ventilated and at a comfortable temperature for the residents as well as the animals. Provide suitable towels for laps as some animals might have accidents while being shown or handled. Each resident should have a towel on his/her lap. Leave the towels in place and take the animal from towel to towel. If staff pick up the towel with the animal, they will be spreading germs from one resident to the next.

Conversation Starters Questions to Handlers:

- Where is your agency geographically located?
- How long has your agency been in existence?
- How is your agency funded?
- How many different species of animals do you have?
- How many animals live there total?
- Can you tell us about the animals you have brought today?
- What unusual characteristics or personality traits do the animals have?

5. More Program Ideas
(Excerpted from *Programs to Remember Unforgettable Pets* by Lynne Martin Erickson.)

... I said earlier that all five senses trigger memories. It's easy to come up with things to look at and listen to and touch that will remind people of pets. It's more difficult to suggest items to taste or smell (unless you can pick up the scent of catnip). The topic of pets has offered fewer than average number of food ideas, but I've buried a couple of them here for you to find. Read on...

Put Together an Intergenerational Group

Even if we have not experienced the intimacy of having a family pet, most of us respond viscerally to animals. "You want to touch them. You want to cuddle them. You want to feed them. You want to play with them. You want to care for them," and, once done, "you're hooked," says Bruce Vogel, author of **Pets and Their People** (1984) in which he reasons that humans are biologically programmed to have pets.

Because this attraction to animal companions seems to be universal, bridging nationalities, cultures, genders and ages, it provides an ideal topic for intergenerational groups. Students and older adults can easily express feelings about pets that span generations. They can investigate together the many topics generated by an interest in animals; and the multisensory nature of your program resources and of animals themselves will appeal to learners with many kinds of abilities. The topic possibly owes its power to the subtlety and significance of human and animal communication, "the closest thing we know to mind reading." claims Jean Craighead George (1985) in **How to Talk to Your Animals**. Whatever the reason, feelings, opinions and information about pets are both personal and profound, a perfect combination for fascinating intergenerational exploration.

Adopt a Pet

I can't help but suggest that you have your group adopt a pet, if you're in a position to do it. A nursing home, retirement complex or housing unit provides a home environment. Phil Arkow (1987) has written a comprehensive step-by-step guide to adopting a pet for a therapy program.

He writes: "Pets provide continual access to uncomplicated affection on demand and are an ice breaking catalyst to group communication and laughter...Animals can trigger reminiscences and cause withdrawn residents to talk about experiences for weeks after a pet-facilitated intervention."

While a dog or cat comes to mind first, there is much entertainment — and discussion — to be gained by adopting a pair of birds in a cage or some fish in a bowl or an aquarium.

At Least Have A Pet Come for A Visit

If full-time pet ownership is more than you and your group want to handle, you still have the option of a visiting pet program. There are a variety of organizations across the country who might help you. A nursing home Activity Director in Norwalk, CA reported that she works with their local Humane Society:

"The Humane Society is very willing to bring the cats and puppies each month. It's a positive experience for all the animals and many of them get placed with staff or residents' families who fall in love with them... We tried having a resident pet, but as 'everybody's pet,' he was largely ignored. In the current arrangement, all the residents look forward to the visits. The animals stay from one to two hours and their coming always prompts reminiscences about former pets. We find we get the greatest response from the most confused patients on our nursing floors. Everyone seems to recognize and relate to animals."

A nursing home in Illinois works with the local Girl Scouts to sponsor an annual pet show for their residents. The combination of children, pets and older people has been a consistent success. The

Scouts organize the show and bring their own pets. They describe their animals to residents and show them off, allowing anyone who's interested to pet them and ask questions. The residents then judge the winners in several categories. According to the Activity Director: "We have everything from dogs to rabbits to gerbils; one year we even had a goat. Because the girls are serious about the contest, they keep good control of the pets. Even the goat was a perfect gentleman."

Your friends and community organizations are your resources to provide variations on the theme. Or write and ask The Delta Society for information on their Pet Partnerships Program (their address is at the end of this chapter). This program provides a national network of registered pet partners available for volunteer visits. These pets have been screened and temperament-tested by a veterinarian or approved trainer, and all dogs have passed the Canine Good Citizen Test.

Sponsor An Animal

Allergic to cats? Afraid of dogs? Hate frogs and fish? Think birds stink? If you live in a community with a zoo, you and your group may be able to "adopt an animal." Many zoos allow groups to nominally adopt one of their animals. In return for donations to the care and feeding of an animal, you can be kept current on what's happening in your animal's corner of the zoo. You might go yourself and take some pictures to display. Your group can choose a name for the animal, learn about him or her and follow the animal's news.

Celebrate National Cat Week

The original National Cat Week was celebrated November 1-7, 1956. Now it's just the first full week in November. Why not make something of it? Adopt a cat. Host a cat show. Hang up some cat cartoons and some posters. Use one (or more) of the many cat books in the resource list to talk about cats throughout history.

Schedule a time for everyone to take a *cat*nap in honor of the occasion. Serve tuna sandwiches. Or sardines. Or make cut-out cookies using a cat cookie cutter. Serve anything with *cat*sup.

Cut out a mouse from hook-and-loop fabric and throw Velcro balls at it. (Or, if your group members are dart throwers, make a mouse dart board.) Play the sound track from the stage production of "Cats." Get the video and show "That Darn Cat." Try to *cat*ch your group members by quizzing them about words that begin with the letters c-a-t.

Lots of things remind people of cats. The catfish has whiskers and the catbird has a cry that sounds like a catcall. The cattails that grow in damp areas have long, fuzzy tips and a marble with a certain kind of glow is called a cat's eye. A catnap is a short snooze and a narrow place to cross, often high in the air, is a catwalk.

Don't Forget National Dog Week

When I called our local librarian to ask the dates for National Dog Week, she told me that every week is dog week at her house, but the official designation is the last full week in September. So, celebrate! Adopt a dog. Host a dog show. Hang up some Snoopy cartoons. Get art prints from the library. Read dog stories from the books on the resource list. Serve hot *dog*s (with or without *cat*sup). Or hush puppies. Or make cut-out cookies using a dog cookie cutter. Cut out a dog from a hook-and-loop fabric and throw Velcro balls at it. Or make a dog dart board. Get the video and show "Lassie," or "Old Yeller," or "The Shaggy Dog." Invite a dog trainer to speak to your group. Or better yet, arrange a field trip to an obedience school. (If you live in St. Louis, visit the Dog Museum at 1721 South Madison.) Get someone to do a demonstration of "walking the dog" with a yo-yo.

Familiarity breeds popularity. Talk about breeds of dogs that people have owned through the years. Make a chart.

6. Programs To Remember Unforgettable Pets
by Lynne Martin Erickson

Animals make people happier, healthier and more sociable. The pet owners and former pet owners in your discussion groups will have much to say about the animals they have known and loved: their names, physical characteristics, cute tricks and services provided. Every pet is special to its owner.

People will talk about how good their pets have made them feel. The devoted companionship of a loyal dog or the contented purring of an affectionate cat can give more comfort than most tonics. In your groups there will be tales of devotion about animals who met their owners at the door each day and some who brought slippers or papers. There will be reports of heroism regarding dangers thwarted and children found. There will be all kinds of stories about all kinds of pets.

And there will be sadness about pets who have died and are very much missed. It is as important for people to be able to share their sad memories as their happy ones. According to Myrna Solganick, a psychotherapist with Affiliated Counseling Services in Madison, Wisconsin, it is important to talk about the loss of a beloved animal and not just put it aside. "Unlike a human death that is attended to by certain traditions, there are no rituals to attend to when a pet dies. Religion may not be a comfort." She goes on to explain that "Pets give us unconditional love. They are like children that never grow up. They always need us. Their death leaves us with feelings of helplessness, with feelings that we could have done more. It is never too late to resolve those feelings of grief and guilt."

There will be people in your group who have never had pets of their own. This does not necessarily mean that they will have nothing to say on the subject. They may share memories of other people's pets. Or they may talk about why they never had a pet or why they would never want one!

Prompting Memories And Discussion

The longer you spend programming on the topic of pets, the more opportunities you offer for people to become involved. A single program goes by quickly and many people won't be able to call up their memories or stories without a chance to think more about them. Separate programs with some time in between allow people to chat with their families and friends independently on the topic. Perhaps a family member can find a picture or other memento for your group member to share.

All five senses trigger memories. In any group, but especially older adults who have had sight and hearing losses, often the more senses you involve in your programming, the more people you are able to involve in your programming, and the more completely you are able to involve them. Bring in things to touch (pet toys, leashes, collars, imitation fur, cages), to look at, to pass around and to talk about.

Discuss One Topic At A Time

The topics below suggest the variety of directions in which your reminiscing about pets can be led. Use just one for single session or choose two or three and put them together. Choose resources to go along with each topic: pictures to look at, music to listen to, things to touch or stories and poems to read.

You might begin your first session by asking who has had a pet or perhaps asking the name and kind of pet that was the favorite of each of your group members. You might make a list tallying how many of which kinds of pets have been owned by your members or what kind of pets were their favorites. That way people will know from the beginning that your program is not for spectators only.

Our Family Pet

Did your family have a pet when you were growing up? Who took care of it? Did you have a pet when your children were growing up? Did your pet have a favorite among your family members?

In what family activities did your pet participate? Did you have a family photo taken with your pet? If so, do you still have a copy? Tell about it. (Or bring it to the next group meeting, if you can!)

How We Got Our Pets

Where did you get the pets who became members of your family? Do you know an unusual story about how a pet joined the family?

What were the names of the pets in your family? How did they get their names? What pet names have you heard that were interesting?

Pets and Children

Which do you think are easier to raise: pets or children? Why? What are the advantages of having pets and children at the same time? What are the disadvantages?

Do you think goldfish make good pets? Why or why not? Have you ever had goldfish? Would you like to have a bowl of goldfish?

Pets are Not for Children Only

What are the advantages of human companionship over animal companionship? What are the advantages of animal friends over human ones?

This short poem was written in 1928 by Sir Alexander Gray, a Scottish professor and poet:

On a Cat Aging
He blinks upon the hearth-rug
And yawns in deep content,
Accepting all the comforts
That Providence has sent.

Louder he purrs and louder,
In one glad hymn of praise
For all the night's adventures,
For quiet, restful days.
Life will go on forever,
With all that cat can wish;
Warmth and the glad procession
Of fish and milk and fish.
Only — the thought disturbs him —
He's noticed once or twice,
That times are somehow breeding
A nimbler race of mice.

How is a cat aging like a person aging? How is it different?
What do you notice changing with the times?

Rx: Pets

Daily care and feeding is one of the major components of
having a pet. What is good about this for children? For adults? For
older adults? What is difficult about this for children? For adults?
For older adults?

The Down Side

What are the disadvantages of pet ownership? Do you think
they outweigh the advantages?

Have you held burial services, funerals or had memorials for
pets that you have had? Tell about them. (How old were you?
What did you do?)

Do you think that pets should be allowed in parks? What rules
would you suggest? Should cats be kept on leashes when they're
outside? Should dogs?

Do you agree that the pain of losing a pet is never greater than
the joy of having had one? What are the joys of having a pet?

"My Dog's Bigger Than Your Dog"

Think about just one of your family pets. What was it that made that pet special? What was best about it or what was it best at doing? Why did you choose that pet to think about?

What tricks have you trained your pets to do? What are the most unusual tricks you have ever seen a pet do?

What is your advice for someone who is thinking about getting a pet?

Remember A Book about a Memorable Animal

Take another look at some of the animal stories you and your group members enjoyed as children (or parents). Read them together or enjoy a video of one that has been made into a movie. Here's a list to get you started, along with the years they were written.

Black Beauty (1877)   The Jungle Book (1894)
Call of the Wild (1903)   The Wind in the Willows (1907)
Lad: A Dog (1919)   Winnie-the-Pooh (1926)
Lassie, Come Home (1940)   My Friend Flicka (1941)
The Black Stallion (1941)   Misty of Chincoteague (1933)
National Velvet (1949)   Charlotte's Web (1952)
Old Yeller (1956)   The Incredible Journey (1961)
Rascal (1963)

Create A Memorial

The Tenth Good Thing About Barney by Judith Viorst (1971) was written for children. But the thought behind it is for people of all ages and that's just the first of many good things about this story. Barney was a cat who died. This story is about how a little boy who loved him manages to live with that. He begins by having a funeral and trying to come up with ten good things about Barney. This is a wonderful way to memorialize a cat, dog, bird or any other friend.

After listening to the story, group members may want to make their own lists of ten good things about their own pets. Or they may want to talk about other good ways they have memorialized their pets (or other friends) who have died.

Help people to memorialize the pets they have loved by sharing their thoughts and memories and perhaps by preserving them in some way. Some options are a story, poem, artwork, a skit or something as short as an epitaph. You might get your group started with this one from Lord Byron, who wrote it to be inscribed on a monument to his Newfoundland dog:

> *Near this spot are deposited the remains of one who possessed Beauty without Vanity, Strength without Insolence, Courage without Ferocity and all Virtues of Man, without his Vices. This Praise, which would be unmeaning Flattery if inscribed over human ashes, is but a just tribute to the Memory of Boatswain, a Dog.*

Save Those Memories! Hang a Gallery

Because pets appeal strongly to the visual sense, take advantage of the photographs you can find for displays and discussion. Collect snapshots and personal videocassettes: create a bulletin board, photo album or cassette corner based on family pet or animal experiences.

Ask group members to illustrate with animals their poems, essays and stories (or those written by others). Create sculptures of animals (real or fantastic) from clay, Playdough or papier-mâché. Make animal masks to display or parade.

Cut photographs and other graphics from magazines and make an animal collage, a jigsaw-type puzzle or an illustrated calendar. Create an animal mural on butcher paper or a hall wall.

Finally...

I hope that you have seen by now that there are many ways to prompt memories and stories of pets, up to and including the use of a real live pet. Our non-profit corporation has produced and packaged a variety of reminiscence program for older adults. Family pets are irresistible memory triggers for seniors as illustrated by a nursing home resident who was moved to tell the tale of her Persian kitten, Lord Ruffles II. "I remember so well his formal name, but I called him Dickey Boy," the program participant recollected. "I dressed him up in doll clothes and took him out on carriage rides. When the poor cat finally died, the manager of my father's factory made a casket for Dickey Boy. It was a cold winter and it was too cold to dig into the yard. Many family members and friends mourned Dickey Boy and we had a perpetual funeral in the garage 'til spring." Clearly, the unconditional love and devotion of pets make them a pleasurable topic for remembering.

As other Bi-Folkal kits, *Remembering Pets* provides a wealth of resources for anyone working with older adults. In addition to 80 slides and accompanying narrative tape, the kit includes a second tape which is equally suitable for dog and cat lovers alike. Side one consists of sing-along songs (including, of course, "How Much Is That Doggie In The Window." Side two features cat tales and ends with a discussion of whether or not cats are people. Supplemental activities Paws for Pictures (12 large black and white photos with discussion-starter questions) and skits (complete with dog and cat masks) make excellent program-starters. The kits also contain multiple copies of Reigning Cats and Dogs, a booklet of large print songs, poems and quotations as well as a unique bag of tricks called "parafurnalia" with imitation Dalmatian fur, lamb's wool and even a grooming comb. The accompanying program manual contains, in addition to a discussion of memory-sharing and tips on program planning, a list of resources available in libraries, discussion-starter questions and ideas for spin-off activities.

Remembering Pets is a treasure for those involved in program-planning for older adults. What better topic for reminiscing than family pets?

Resources

The Delta Society. They are the national organization dedicated to improving the interactions of people, animals and the environment and they are a wonderful resource available to you. They sent us a folder stuffed with articles and ideas together with a list of additional material to order and audiovisual resources for rental or purchase. Write to The Delta Society at 289 Perimeter Road East, Renton, WA 98055-1329 or call (800) 869-6898 or fax at (425) 235-1076.

Dogs & Their Women by Barbara Cohen and Louise Taylor (Little, Brown, 1989). This is a collection of photographs together with reminiscences like this one which accompanies a black-and-white photo of an older woman with a little furry white dog. "Toby went everywhere with me…I buried him with a special stone in my back yard. The forget-me-nots come up every year. I've adopted a stray cat and I started to collect Teddy bears, but it's Toby I really miss." There are lots more and every one is a discussion starter.

How to Start a Pet Therapy Program: A Guideline for Health Care Professionals by Phil Arkow. In this 32 page booklet, Arkow details the steps of meeting with the administration, planning with your group members, contacting the families and making all necessary decisions before the animal is brought into the group. Order your copy by sending $6.00 (including shipping) to Phil Arkow, 37 Hillside Road, Stratford, NJ 08084. Phone: 609-627-5118, fax 609-627-2252, e-mail, arkowpets@aol.com.

Pets & Patients: Therapy That Works. The Journal of Long Term Care Administration. American College of Health Care Administrators, vol. 12, no. 4; winter 1984. This special issue includes a discussion of "why this human-animal interaction is so therapeutic in nursing homes and a systematic needs assessment survey for determining whether your facility would benefit from this program."

Pets and the Elderly: The Therapeutic Bond. Haworth Press, 1984. Originally an issue of Activities, Adaptions and Aging, this volume is a reference for therapists working with older adults. It covers a variety of issues relating to pet visitation programs and pets in residence.

Remembering Pets. Bi-Folkal Productions, 1991. A complete multi-media, multi-sensory program kit of reminiscence resources on the topic of pets. For more information about this kit and 15 others, contact Bi-Folkal at 809 Williamson Street, Madison, WI 53703 (608) 251-2818.

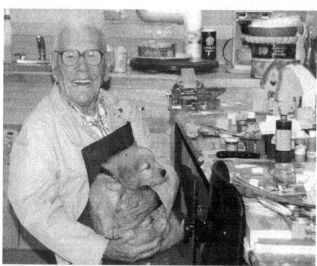

John Baxter takes a moment out from his crafts project to say hello to Nickie.

Chapter 5

Pet Therapy Survey

Pet Therapy Survey Coding

A survey was conducted concerning the makeup of existing pet therapy programs. Twenty-one responses were received from a questionnaire that was circulated at state and national workshops and conventions in the Spring of 1990. Although this is not a sufficient number to yield any statistically significant data, it does provide some interesting information about the experiences people have typically had in implementing programs of this sort. The following is a compilation of these twenty-one surveys.

Duration of Program: The length of time the programs had been implemented ranged from 2-15 years, with the average being 6 years.

Facility Population: The population of the facilities ranged from 15-330, averaging 134 people per facility.

Levels of Care: Multiple levels of care were represented, from adolescent through elderly, including intermediate, skilled, short and long term, assisted and independent living, cerebral palsy, multiple sclerosis and mental health care.

Types of Animal Programs: Over 75% of the responding facilities had a visiting pet program.

About half the facilities kept at least one kind of furry animal (cat, dog, rabbit) in residence. With or without a furry pet in residence, many programs used a combination of plush animals, fish, birds and/or visiting animals.

In terms of number of therapies established at each facility, one third of the facilities had one type of pet therapy program, one third used two forms, a quarter used three forms and two of the facilities had four kinds of pet therapy available.

One third of the facilities kept dogs, making them the most popular choice. Nearly a third kept fish. One quarter made use of plush animals. Rabbits, birds and cats were each resident at two facilities apiece.

Dog breeds included: Toy Poodle, Golden Retriever, Miniature Schnauzer, leader dogs, Sheltie, Labrador and Peek-a-Poo.

Reasons for Implementation of Program:
a) Therapeutic Value:
- The therapeutic value of having pets was recognized
- Benefits seen in other nursing homes
- Information on value obtained from workshop and consultant
- Responsiveness of those who are generally unresponsive
- Animals get through the "dementia fog"
- Unrestricted love between humans and animals
- Stuffed "pets" in residents' rooms stimulated sharing experiences

b) Requests/Personal interest:
- Activity Director's own enjoyment of animals
- Love of animals displayed by recreational therapy staff
- Suggestion from administration
- Resident council asked to have dogs and cats visit the facility
- Interest expressed by residents
- Residents spoke of their pets in reminiscence sessions

c) Opportunity:
- A professional dog trainer volunteered to introduce a program
- Toy poodle, with a nice personality, found on street
- Stray dog was brought to the facility
- Visiting dogs were volunteered by their owners
- Rabbits were donated

How the Program was Implemented:

a) Pet visits:
- Staff member brought in the first animal
- 4-H club visits
- Local kennel club
- Pet store
- Humane society
- "Pet show" organized
- Families asked to bring in pets
- Volunteers brought in visiting pets

b) Resident pets:
- Local shelter
- Pet store
- Dog donated by kennel
- Homeless puppy appeared at facility

Sources of Support:

a) In-house:
1. Staff:
   - Administration
   - Medical Director
   - Supervisor
   - Nursing Department, Director of Nurses
   - Environmental Services staff
2. Volunteers:
   - Women's Auxiliary
   - Board of Directors
3. Residents and Families

b) Outside:
  * Veterinarians
  * 4-H clubs
  * Red Cross

Program Goals:
  a) Reminiscence:
   * To reach patients who identify with pets from the past
   * To bring back memories of having pets
   * To provide reminiscence opportunities
  b) Emotional/Cognitive:
   * To provide unconditional love/affection by residents
   * To allow all residents to express feelings of love and caring
   * To stimulate appropriate conversation from confused residents
  c) Physical/Tactile:
   * To provide opportunities for exercise
   * To hold something living and small
  d) Social:
   * To provide programming for room-bound residents
   * To increase resident's socialization
   * To provide interaction between the community and residents
   * To provide interaction between frail elderly and pets
   * To bring cheer and life to patients/residents
   * To allow each animal time to spend with each resident
  e) Operational:
   * To reinstate the 4-H kennel club program
   * To continue/expand the program
   * To continue to have a resident take care of an animal
   * To create a more home-like atmosphere for the facility

Program Benefits:
  * Response from those who are ordinarily confused, uninterested

- Increased verbalization
- Love shown by residents unable to express in other ways
- Unconditional love provided by animals
- Respond to soft and cuddly animals (stuffed or live)
- Smiles and happiness
- Calming effect on upset, loud residents
- Making residents feel special and needed
- Provision of a sense of usefulness and self-esteem
- Memory recall and sharing of residents' past pets
- Something to look forward to
- In-room enjoyment from visiting animals
- Room-bound residents come out to see the pets

Problems Experienced: Most facilities reported no problems, but the following are the ones encountered by some facilities:

a) Animal Behavior:
   - Some animals did not mingle well
   - Occasional noises that scared cats
   - Housebreaking pets
   - Bunnies ran free in Activity Room and got into everything
   - Changes in living arrangements for the pet (traumatic for pet)

b) Animal Upkeep:
   - Finding someone to care for live-in pets on the weekends
   - Keeping crates clean

c) Animal/Human Interactions:
   - Overfeeding or inappropriate feeding of animals
   - Keeping animals away from residents that were afraid of them
   - Some residents did not want animals around
   - Finding out which residents do not care to visit with pets
   - Some staff and residents allergic to cats
   - Avoiding pet injury from wheelchairs

d) Program:
   - Cancellations of volunteers program
   - Not enough visits
   - Occasional families who did not approve of the program

What would be done differently: Most respondents said they would not make any changes if they were to start over. The few changes (aside from "start the program sooner") that were suggested fell into roughly three categories:

a) Do better planning:
   - More careful planning before the animal arrives
   - Have a play pen first
   - A check of residents' likes/dislikes for animals
   - Choose an older cat so that personality could be evaluated before bringing it into the facility
   - Estimate costs better to avoid cost overruns of as much as several hundred dollars
b) Institute feeding controls:
   - Closer supervision for residents who try to feed the animals
   - Signs made ahead of time asking residents not to feed animals
c) Create a larger program:
   - Have more frequent visits and with more animals
   - Encourage more participants to come in
   - Have more volunteers so cancellations can be covered

Program Summaries

The following summaries are a sample of the completed surveys received, arranged to reflect some of the variations on pet therapy that have been tried.

Dogs

Menorah Park, Beechwood, Ohio

This 330 bed facility of highly skilled residents has had a pet therapy program for about two and a half years. It is centered around Heather, a female Golden Retriever. Nathalie Diener, Director of Recreational Therapy, reported that this breed was chosen after much research including talking with veterinarians, animal lovers and other facilities with pets and reading about the subject.

Heather is supervised by one of the recreational therapy staff members each day that she is in the facility. That person is responsible for all of Heather's needs during the day. Although Heather started out at Menorah Park five days a week, she is now shared by a sister facility for two of the five days that she provides therapy. The goal is for every resident to be visited by Heather each week. As reported by so many others, these visits have led to increased resident verbalization while they are petting her and evident pleasure on their faces when she is around them.

Heather is taken home at night and on the weekends by a staff person, but this has not been easy. She is currently in her third home and this has been very hard on her. If implementing this program today this is the only area that Ms. Diener would change. That is, she would have made more concrete arrangements for Heather's care away from the home before starting the program.

The Evergreens, Moorestown, New Jersey

Donna Loftus, Activity Director, has a program in place that provides therapy for her 116 long-term care residents. A sheltie named Lady has lived at the home for the past six years, having come to the facility fully trained. There have been no problems as Lady just blended in as if she had always been there. She is well-behaved and loves the residents as well as the many children who visit the facility. Lady sleeps in the room of a resident, who is also responsible for her daily walking, feeding and brushing. The home provides a budget for veterinarian bills, licensing and grooming.

One of the residents is also responsible for taking Lady to visit through the nursing care unit at least once every day. Lady is kept on a leash for these visits and the resident who escorts her is always sure to knock on the door and gain permission before entering a resident's room. Ms. Loftus notes that regressed residents "light-up" when they see Lady and enjoy petting her and touching her soft fur.

One problem that has been experienced with the program is that the residents bring scraps from the dining room table to share with Lady. Her subsequent weight gain was quickly solved by putting up signs that read "Please don't feed Lady."

The Evergreens also has a visiting pet program in which a local animal farm, for a small donation, brings pets to visit. Usually thirty to thirty-five residents are in attendance for their one hour visit.

A unique Christmas Program was started by Ms. Loftus in 1989. A letter was sent to each residents' family asking for a donation of a teddy bear, to be dressed in a manner that would represent the residents' life-long occupation. Many families responded, some with bears, some with financial support. For those residents without family participation, bears were purchased and dressed with the assistance of staff. The bears were given to each resident on Christmas morning. Increased socialization was noticed immediately and the bears are still seen on many of the residents' beds or somewhere in their rooms. In January a tea was held to which everyone brought their bear and talked about their careers. As this project took a long time to complete, it is Ms. Loftus' recommendation that it be started by early October at the latest.

Ms. Loftus believes that pet therapy is a wonderful program for all of her residents and is sure that Lady will have a successor when that time comes.

Cats

Birchwood Care Center, Marne, Michigan

Birchwood Care Center provides basic, skilled and foster care for 197 residents. Their pet therapy program has been in place for four years and was started because of the love of animals displayed by the recreational therapy staff and the expressed interest of the residents. Current goals include providing physical and emotional stimulation.

Although several families bring in dogs to visit with the residents, the program mainly revolves around two cats. They came to the facility as kittens and were given all the necessary shots, neutered and declawed. Litter boxes were placed in the Activity Office and in another location in the building where the kittens often frequent. The cats live in the Activity Room but they have the freedom to roam the halls. They also are taken by the recreation staff to do one-to-one visits on a regular basis. Some residents are allergic to the cats, but these residents were moved to rooms where the cats do not visit.

It is the feeling of the recreational therapy staff that live-in pets help to make the facility more like home and that families are happy to see them there. Cats were chosen because they are easier to care for. Staff time is not required to take them outside and they can stay alone on the weekends.

The benefits of this program are many: residents who do not routinely respond smile when they feel the cats fur and hear them purr. Those who rarely smile or who show little interest in company often respond when one of the cats comes for a visit. Other residents who are able to get around on their own actually plan their schedule around visits with the cats in the office area. They also love to brag about the cats following them through the hallways or sitting on their beds.

Jill Hausmann, CTRS, now feels, however, that if the program were to be started over, adult cats should be chosen as their personalities can be more accurately predicted. Another problem noted and one certainly not exclusive to this facility, is that the cats are over nourished and have become "fat cats." This has necessitated their being locked up on Sundays when no recreation staff are available to prevent the weekend staff from feeding them goodies.

Rabbits

Shore Haven Living Center, Grand Haven, Michigan

This 126 bed skilled facility has had a pet therapy program in place for approximately three years. Kristine Larsen, acting on the suggestion of her consultant, began the program by gaining the support of other department heads and the resident council.

Because their facility is on a busy street, a cat or dog was not considered suitable. A parakeet and fish were tried earlier but had not proved very successful. Because it could be housed in a cage and yet was large enough to be held by the residents, the decision was made to try a rabbit. Costs have been minimal; also families help by bringing in cash donations, as well as carrots, parsley and special rabbit treats.

"Ra-berta" the rabbit, accompanies Ms. Larsen on one-to-one visits. Stuffed animals are also used in one-to-one programming to provide tactile stimulation, but mostly the residents come to see her. Ra-berta makes ten to twenty room visits regularly and another fifteen to twenty residents come to the Activity Room to visit her. Residents are asked upon admission to the facility how they feel about pets and about their animal preferences. If the resident does not want to see any type of pet, it is so noted on their precautions list.

As in other facilities, residents showed affection towards Ra-berta by feeding her donuts, so a sign was soon posted requesting that everyone not feed her. Ms. Larsen suggests that if you are considering a rabbit, make sure that their cage is large enough, that a confined area is available for them to run around in and that they can be taken outside occasionally, either in the cage or in a confined area. Also keep in mind that their cages require frequent cleaning; Ra-berta's cage is cleaned two times a week, with the assistance of residents.

Families and residents get much enjoyment from Ra-berta and she seems to enjoy entertaining them. Stimulation and sharing of memories of past pets, providing something small and living to hold and the expression of feelings of love and caring are some of the benefits that have been derived. Ra-berta has been a great influence on many of the residents since her arrival: eyes twinkle, smiles appear on faces, residents who are withdrawn talk to her and residents who are confused are often able to remember her name and where she lives.

Luther Manor, Saginaw, Michigan

Both bunnies and visiting dogs are used in the pet therapy at this ninety-eight bed skilled nursing care facility. The dogs had been coming in for over two years and the live-in bunnies were introduced in March of 1990.

The administrator, always open to innovative programming, quickly gave his support when the program was suggested. Helen Blood, Activity Director at Luther Manor, got both bunnies from families who were moving and unable to take the bunnies with them. They were accepted by the home with the understanding that if they did not work out, the previous owner would then find other homes for them. The male is six years old and neutered; the female is almost two years old; both are paper trained and live in a six-sided play pen without a floor.

Team work is all important in this program. The dietary staff provides lettuce three times a week which a resident picks up and feeds to the rabbits. The ward clerk, who loves animals, also helps; she is usually the one who cleans up after them. The rabbits enjoy buttered toast and the Activity Director brings each of them a half a piece most mornings. Some of the families bring in fruit, but, as in other facilities, it has become necessary to put up a sign asking that they not be fed by others, as it is difficult to know what they have had.

The bunnies can also be fed by means of a plastic feeding container which can be filled and lasts a long time. It has been Ms. Blood's experience that bunnies are very curious animals and will get into all kinds of things if they are left to run freely, so a pen is advisable. She also expressed concern about odors and the fact that they are somewhat messy, often lying down in their litter box. However, they have brought much pleasure to the residents, many of whom bring their families to see them.

A volunteer also brings her dog Midnight, a small black cocker, to the facility on a weekly basis. The visits are listed on the calendar and the volunteer goes from room to room. She was accompanied by Ms. Blood on her first several visits, but now she goes on her own, making notes of whom she visits and their reactions. She visits about thirty residents in their rooms each week, plus those that are in the halls. Midnight brings much enjoyment to those residents who do not like to leave their rooms and the staff benefit from seeing the pleasure of the residents.

Ms. Blood has also had positive experiences with birds and fish in another facility. It was her feeling, however, that although birds can be dirty, they are less likely to be overfed than fish and can be left enough food for several days. They also are nice for the residents to watch and talk to.

Low Maintenance

Wyomissing Lodge, Reading, Pennsylvania

At this skilled nursing facility, Barbara Mills uses both live and stuffed animal therapy with her 100 residents. A teddy bear tea, where conversation revolves around children, grandchildren and past and present experiences is just one of the animal-centered activities that is held in this facility.

Pet visits are provided by Red Cross volunteers and family members and kittens and puppies are brought in from the Humane Society on a monthly basis. The volunteers are always accompanied by a member of the Activity Staff who oversees the visit in each room. There is also an on-site aquarium which is maintained by the Activity Staff and is a focal point in the activity area.

The current goals for the program include providing programming for residents on bedrest and stimulation for those who identify with pets from the past. Ms. Mills contends that animals have been the only thing that has succeeded in reaching some of the residents. Stuffed animals seem to provide a great source of contentment for certain individuals. They seem to respond to something soft and cuddly, as well as the shared memories.

The only problems associated with this program have occurred when volunteers have had to cancel. On those occasions the staff have tried to compensate, as well as possible, by bringing in their own pets.

Michigan Christian Home, Grand Rapids, Michigan

Pam Spalding, Activity Director for seventy-nine residents, began her program in January of 1988. It includes visits from birds, cats, dogs, rabbits and baby chicks. Ms. Spalding believes that animals bring out a responsiveness that is rarely seen in these residents so she started bringing her own baby kitten to the facility.

The facility has an enclosed patio where her two cats are now brought every two weeks. They are also taken to the residents, who are able to hold, pet and talk to them. In the spring birds and bunnies are borrowed from pet stores and put in a common area where residents can visit them. They, too, are also taken around for one-to-one visits. A deposit is required by the pet store until the animals are safely returned. Baby chicks are obtained in the same manner at Easter time.

In addition, a member of the Humane Society brings in a dog two to three times per month and a western day, when farm animals were brought in by 4-H clubs, has been held.

The primary goal of all these programs is to bring cheer to the residents. (Although the animals seem to be equally enjoyed by the staff!) As many others have noted, the biggest reward is to witness the responses of the residents who are confused and generally unresponsive. Ms. Spalding reports that her biggest problem was when one of her cats got scared, hid under a bed and they were unable to find her for a while. If she were to enhance or change the program in any way, she would do so by having more animals come in and more frequently.

Multiple Therapies

St. Lawrence Dimondale Nursing Center, Dimondale, Michigan

Chris Simons is Activity Director here for one hundred and seventy-eight residents. The pet therapy program has been in existence for six years and was initiated by the administrator. It began with fish, then cats and dogs were added. The cat and fish live at the facility, while the dogs are brought in by the administrator each day. The dogs are taken to residents on bedrest two times a week for special visits.

Newborn farm animals are also brought to the facility (after a tarp is put on the floor) and residents really seem to enjoy seeing this new life. Visitors bring horses to the outside of the center and talk about their history and care. Those residents who can't get out to see them often watch through their windows.

Like so many other facilities, residents at St. Lawrence enjoy feeding the dogs, but this problem has been solved by supervising the dogs more closely. The only other problem reported involved younger dogs biting children when not kept on a leash.

The most enjoyable aspect of the program has been to see the friendships established between the residents and the dogs. Benefits include residents, who otherwise do not respond to anything, responding to the dogs and seeing smiles that are only induced by the animals. The goals of the program are to provide unconditional love, smiles, exercise and reminiscence opportunities.

Conclusions

Although each setting has unique and distinctive characteristics, pet therapy may well be one of the most universal and flexible programs that can be implemented in any facility. The responsiveness of the residents to these programs was mentioned in every survey that was returned.

Which program is right for you? Only you can make that decision. And just maybe there is another yet to be created. Be imaginative: design a program that fits your budget, schedule, resident needs and resources available.

Whatever type of pet therapy program is decided upon, the following guidelines should prove helpful:

- Only embark on this program if you are a true believer in the therapeutic value of pet therapy.
- Gain support from the top. Don't waste time on a program that will not be approved by your administration. Round up other department heads to be your advocates in this endeavor.
- Be explicit in setting up your policies and procedures. Stay within the guidelines of your local and state governments. Take time to plan your pets' schedules *on paper* before you get them. (See examples in *Appendix*.) Inform staff of the pending program and gain their support. Remember, some people are afraid of and/or allergic to animals. Your entire staff may not be able to handle the animal chosen. Be flexible — alternative plans might be needed.
- Be realistic when setting up time frames for implementation of your program.
- Visiting pets require a big commitment from their owners. Obedience training and grooming take large amounts of time. Be prepared to accept changes as they might occur: 4-H'ers go off to college; therapy dog owners move or take on other responsibilities that may keep them from visiting.

- Introducing a live-in pet requires an adjustment period for all concerned. Even completely trained adult dogs need time to learn about their new surroundings, their boundaries and where to go for toileting. Puppies take three years to mature and settle down. The "terrible twos" is a phase that not just human offspring go through — it can be a troublesome time for animals as well.

- Keep in mind that, when selecting a puppy, kitten or bunny that seems very quiet, its adult personality may be quite different. When selecting an adult animal, try to find out as much about its background as possible, including who owned the animal and why it was given up.

- Stand behind your research and convictions about the program. As with any program you create, do the very best that you can, but be prepared for those helpful folks who always know "a better way." Be open to suggestions and ideas but don't become uncertain about the program you have researched and developed. Take suggestions under advisement and research the area again before making any changes.

Perhaps most importantly of all, always keep in mind the welfare of your animals. Remember, they are now totally dependent on you for their upkeep and care. They have rights that need to be considered and you are their primary caregiver.

Chapter 6

Plush/Stuffed Animals

At times, the best choice of a therapy animal may be a stuffed one! There are a few drawbacks that accompany live animal programs. Some facilities may find it difficult or impossible to implement such programs. Certainly they require much in the way of planning, paperwork, personnel and maintenance. In addition, some residents and/or staff may be allergic, afraid or unfamiliar with the special needs of pets. A live pet therapy program may not be the best one with which to begin, or may need augmenting. There are often good reasons to consider the use of plush animal therapy using stuffed animals or dolls.

It is certainly much easier to use stuffed animals rather than live ones. The benefits include having only one initial cost and being required to do much less preparation, paperwork, supervision and maintenance. These "pets" don't even require a license! This type of therapy can run pretty much on its own. The use of small groups, usually centered on reminiscence, can be set up to enhance the program.

It is true that there has been little written about the therapeutic use of stuffed animals with older adults. However, the personal experience of Activity Professionals indicates that they often bring positive responses from residents and have been extremely worthwhile in many programs. The increased socialization is itself a reason to implement such a program.

One study that was done (with forty residents in a long-term care facility) did show some significant results. (Francis and Baly, 1986) Twenty-two of the residents were allowed to choose a plush animal from a group that was presented to them. (The other eighteen were the control group.) Those with the animals named them, carried them around and showed them to visitors. When the residents, who had been pre-tested at the start of the study, were tested again eight weeks later, those who had been given the animals showed significant changes in psychological well-being, social reaction, mental function, life satisfaction, psychological function and level of depression The control group remained unchanged in these areas. Three other tested variables (healthy self-concept, social competence and physical neatness) were apparently unaffected by the possession of the stuffed animal. Francis and Baly summarized their results by stating that "apparently, having a new stimulus which is pleasurable to look at, touch, own and talk about makes a difference — a big difference — even when that something is a plush animal."

A second study (Francis and Munjus, 1988) was undertaken to determine if self-selected plush animals would be accepted by male residents and if the same results as the previous study would be obtained. The males had no trouble accepting the animals and, once again, significant changes were noted in the same variables as listed above. However, the researchers were unable to determine the reasons for these changes. They did conclude that plush animal therapy was a practical, easy and cost-effective approach to therapy.

Finally, a third report (Koedel and Brunecz, 1989) attested to the success of talking baby dolls with patients with Alzheimer's. Unlike the plush animals, they were not left with the residents, but used in supervised sensory stimulation sessions. Fears that these residents would confuse the dolls with real babies were quickly alleviated as the residents not only responded appropriately, but used more complex sentences than usual and demonstrated increased attention spans.

If the decision is made to use stuffed animals or dolls, the following tips on implementing such a program might prove helpful:

1. Gain approval from your administrator or supervisor. Try to determine what the feelings of staff and families are toward

the use of stuffed animals and dolls. Some people have objected to their use because of concerns that they are not age-appropriate. Your program is doomed to failure if those who are to be involved are not convinced of its therapeutic value. I personally believe that the success of any program depends on meeting the residents' needs at the level on which they are able to function.

2. Shop around for the best prices and determine if your budget will allow such a program. Try to find a sponsor (foundation, church or volunteer group) that might donate funds or the stuffed animals themselves.

3. Before purchasing, either make a list of animals available and ask the residents what they would like to have OR make the selection yourself and take the animals on a cart to the residents and allow them to choose the one they want.

4. As in all new programs, inform staff members working in other disciplines about what you are doing and what you hope to achieve. Making them aware of the benefits to the residents will allow them to assist you in making the program work.

5. If you can discreetly tag each animal/doll with one of the resident's name tags used for their clothing, it may be of great help in identifying the animals if they are separated from the resident at any time or for any reason.

6. Make sure that all animals and dolls used are washable and fire retardant.

Below are two suppliers of wonderful plush animals.

The Puppet Petting Zoo
213 Crystal Lake Road, Talland, CT 06084, (203) 872-6899

Carolyn Cook
5 Helm Turn, Willingboro, NJ 08046, (609) 877-6504

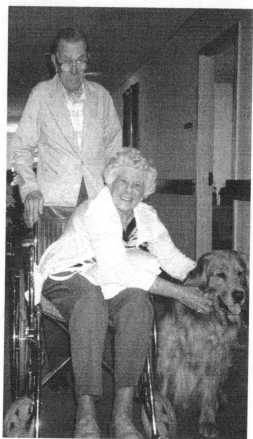

It's never too much trouble for Alice and William Drecks to stop for a visit with Nickie as they travel through the halls of the Masonic Home of New Jersey.

Chapter 7

Dogs

Despite stiff competition from cats, rabbits, fish, birds and, in recent years, potbellied pigs, goats and chinchillas, the most popular choice of a therapy animal remains the dog.

For this reason, this chapter on dogs is the largest and most comprehensive of the chapters in this book. The chapter itself has been divided into three sections, each devoted to a different aspect of dealing with dogs who live and/or work in a long-term care facility.

Section 1: Therapeutic Uses: stories and guidelines relating to the therapeutic work done by dogs.
Section 2: Behavior and Training: understanding and training your dog
Section 3: Policies and Procedures: tips on introducing a puppy and providing day-to-day maintenance of a facility puppy/dog.

With patience, humor and a bit of information, you will be able to establish effective routines and foster the development of deeply satisfying relationships between your therapy dog and both residents and staff.

Senator Vest's Tribute to A Dog

This eloquent tribute to a dog was made during the trial of a man who had shot a neighbor's foxhound. Senator Vest asked for $200 in damages, but after two minutes deliberation the jury awarded $500.

Gentlemen of the jury: The best friend a man has in this world may turn against him and become his enemy. His son or daughter that he has reared with loving care may prove ungrateful. Those who are nearest and dearest to us, those whom we trust with our happiness and our good name, may become traitors to their faith. The money that a man has he may lose. It flies away from him; perhaps when he needs it most. A man's reputation may be sacrificed in a moment of ill-considered action. The people who are prone to fall on their knees to do us honor when success is with us may be the first to throw the stone of malice when failure settles its cloud upon our heads. The one absolutely unselfish friend that a man can have in this selfish world, the one that never deserts him, the one that never proves ungrateful or treacherous, is his dog.

Gentlemen of the jury, a man's dog stands by him in prosperity and in poverty, in health and in sickness. He will sleep on the cold ground, where the wintry winds blow and the snow drives fiercely, if only he may be near his master's side. He will kiss the hand that has no food to offer. He will lick wounds and sores that come in encounters with the roughness of the world. He guards the sleep of his pauper master as if he were a prince. When all other friends desert, he remains. When riches take wings and reputation falls to pieces, he is as constant in his love as the sun in its journey through the heavens. If fortune drives the master forth an outcast in the world, friendless and homeless, the faithful dog asks no higher privilege than that of accompanying him to guard against danger, to fight against his enemies and, when the last scene of all comes and death takes the master in its embrace and his body is laid away in the cold ground, no matter if all other friends pursue their way, there by his graveside will the noble dog be found, his head between his paws, his eyes sad but open in alert watchfulness, faithful and true even to death.

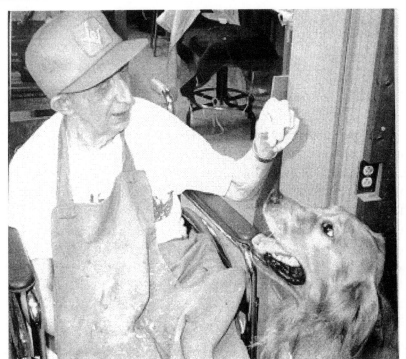

Residents like Bill Stillwell benefit from exercise when feeding and stroking pets like Nicky.

Therapeutic Uses

Working With Therapy Dogs
by Randie Dale Duretz, ADC

My involvement with Pet Therapy began in 1985. My father and my aunt had made the big decision to place my ninety year old Bubba (Jewish grandmother) in a nursing home. Bubba was alert, but very disoriented with respect to people, place and time, and in need of round-the-clock, long-term care. She was hard of hearing, had lost a great deal of weight, needed a wheelchair and had to totally depend on someone escorting her to and from any place that she needed to go.

Bubba became the new resident, one of one hundred and twenty, at the Rivers Edge Nursing and Rehabilitation Center in northeast Philadelphia. Family members visited her daily, but they had a very hard time dealing with the new situation. Bubba was now living in a nursing home: sharing a room with another resident, needing total care after all her years of independence and often not recognizing her loving family.

She had talked in the past, and now in the present, about her mixed breed dog, Blackie, the dog that had lived with her and my Zada (Jewish grandfather). This dog had also helped to man their south Philadelphia butcher shop. She spoke about what a good dog he had been and how they had rewarded him with leftover meat from their shop.

This was where my three collies and I came in. The dogs were: Mazel (the father, who since passed away in 1989), Bagels (the mother) and Kasha, their son. At that time my three lovable, furry, four-legged "kids" weren't certified for Pet Therapy and I knew nothing about the Pet Therapy program. I did, however, receive permission from the administrator to bring the dogs into the facility to visit with my Bubba.

So it began! One night, after putting in a full eight or nine hours with my hundred and forty residents and our fun-filled activity schedule, I groomed the three collies and ran them around in the back yard. Then off we went — accompanied by a bag (packed with doggie treats, a brush, plastic pick-up bags) and a lump in my stomach from not knowing what to expect. I also included a container of water and their bowl for a snack after the visit.

We arrived at the nursing home at 6:15 p.m. The residents had just finished their dinner and were sitting in the hallways and day room. Mazel, Bagels, Kasha and I walked down the long hallway trying to find Bubba's room. We stopped at the second floor nursing station to introduce ourselves and to ask if it was all right for the other residents to touch and visit with the dogs.

We received four-star, A-OK treatment; we were stopped in the hallway by everyone — residents as well as staff members. All that could be heard were the "wows," "ahs," "here comes three Lassie dogs," "I love dogs," "I had a dog," and "can't I see them?" "Sure," I said. "My name is Randie. These are my three best friends and they can be yours also." The interaction between people in this home was just fantastic. I felt something very special going on and thought that possibly there could be even more to this.

After fifteen minutes, I finally made it over to Bubba's room. I peeked in and saw her sitting in her wheelchair — a frail, gray-haired little lady, just looking out her window. We walked into her room and her eyes brightened up. She had a smile on her face and raised her voice. "Lady, bring them over to me," she said. Bubba told me that she had Blackie and that she loved him and all dogs. I knew that she had no idea who I was at the time, but I had to put that sorrow behind me and just remember the good, fond memories. Now I had to have her enjoy these happy moments with my dogs.

Bubba asked me the dogs' names and repeated them after me. She laughed and said, "three Jewish dogs in my room, boy, am I lucky." I did have to speak louder than normal so that she could hear me. She seemed to be in seventh heaven, enjoying the interaction between the dogs. She reminisced about Blackie and enjoyed petting and hugging the dogs, as well as receiving their kisses and their paws. She was very happy with this visit, but still did not know who I was throughout it. I tried not to let it bother me and just let her enjoy the dogs' visit.

When visiting time was over and we had to leave, I gave her a kiss. She said, "Lady, can you bring them back to see me?" I said I would and left. Again, I had that special feeling inside.

Later that night, I opened up a dog magazine and there was an article about pet therapy: "Do you have a friendly, obedience trained dog? Do you enjoy bringing smiles and joy into other people's lives? Then contact Therapy Dogs International. The K-9 Stripers. Dogs with a Purpose." At that time the person to contact was Jack Butrick, President of Therapy Dogs International, based in Cheyenne, Wyoming. This group is now headquartered in California (see *Appendix*). The Butricks started their own therapy group — Therapy Dogs Inc., in Cheyenne.

Dogs who join either of the therapy groups must have an AKC obedience title or a training club graduation certificate. They must also pass the Therapy test and Canine Good Citizen test. The dogs are tested on how they react around gurneys, wheelchairs, walkers and people who yell (a common situation with hard-of-hearing residents/patients).

These dogs must be at least one year of age, well-groomed, clean and parasite free. Their owners must be well-groomed as well. The dogs must have a good temperament and be well-socialized towards other animals and people. They must be in perfect health and must have had all their current shots. (It's a good idea to keep copies of their vaccination records in your wallet and to give them to each home you visit.)

Basic training consists of acquiring a knowledge of commands, including "sit," "down," "heel" and "come" and learning to perform them reliably, even in the face of extreme distractions. The dogs must also become accustomed to working on a variety of surfaces: grass, dirt, asphalt, carpet and linoleum flooring. It is also helpful if they are trained to be at ease while riding in elevators. The registration fee for both Therapy Dogs International and Therapy Dogs, Inc. is very reasonable. For any additional dogs of the owner, there is a small extra charge. Both of these groups provide insurance that covers all legal liability for all Therapy Dog-related activities, provided that there are no fees received for these services.

The handlers/owners receive membership ID cards. The dogs receive tags that attach to their collars. One side reads, "I am a Therapy Dog," while "Registered Therapy Dog, TDI," appears on the other.

Back to my own story. Time passed. I read up on Therapy Dogs. My dogs and I went through the tests and we passed. Mazel, Bagels and Kasha were now ready to start our visits as Certified Therapy Dogs.

Bubba's home was the site of our first visit as certified Therapy Dog volunteers. The residents looked forward to our visits; some marked their calendars and counted the days until the next one. Room-to-room visits were great: a fragile woman sat in her chair by the window with a blanket draped across her lap, looking out. When the dogs and I entered and knocked, the woman's face became "illuminated" and her arms extended to embrace the dogs.

In addition to room visits, we did group visitations. The Activity Professionals would gather the residents into the community and day rooms and I introduced the three collies and myself to about twenty-five people. I told them the names and ages of the dogs and a little about who we were and what we did. I put on a little obedience show, showed the residents how to groom the dogs and even brought along several costumes in which to dress the dogs. We then walked around the room for questions.

These visits didn't stop with Bubba's nursing home. As other homes found out about the three collies and me, we added them, growing to seven homes plus a special visit to a hospital for people who were headed home.

Some of the individuals with whom we work had animals for forty or fifty years of their lives and having dogs around again stirs up positive memories and emotions in them. Research has shown that animals have positive effects on health, emotional well-being and social contacts. Indeed, the best medicine for some mental and physical ailments may not come in a bottle but may be in having contact with a Pet Therapy Dog.

Researchers have shown that interacting with animals can lower blood pressure and heart rate, build confidence and self-esteem, increase mobility, offer security and help elderly nursing home residents by improving verbal communication and encouraging activity.

The Therapy Dogs love their work and look forward to visiting these homes. These dogs don't care about a resident's physical appearance, how he or she smells or what type of disability they may have. Where else can they enjoy so much love, attention and joy in such a short time? A few minutes of being loved and loving a Therapy Dog is so meaningful for an elderly person. For them, it can be the highlight of a long, dreary day.

Residents prominently display pictures that I've taken of them and my dogs on their mirrors and the dressers beside their beds. They buy dog treats for them and celebrate their doggie birthdays. We also get great feedback from family members; I've even been invited to talk to Family Support Groups.

What follows are highlights from some of our visits:

Betty, who used to own a little poodle, looks forward to the dogs' visits. "I love it. Why not? You feel as if you're outside again," she said, while stroking Kasha and letting the dog kiss her chin.

Olga: "Where's my baby?" (The change nurse has gone into the room before we came in, put a sheet on her bed and given her permission to get up on the bed.) This is Kasha's cue to jump on the bed and lay beside her, placing his head on Olga's lap. She leans down towards the gentle and loving collie and prods him for a kiss.

Hugging and talking to him directly in front of his face like a child, she punctuates her comments with a big smile. Olga is usually the last on our rounds, since we can never seem to leave her room.

Mary, a quiet lady who hadn't spoken for three months, was waiting in her geri-chair. Bagels and I approached and Bagels put her front paws up on the chair. At that, Mary yelled out "Get your G-D dog off my chair!" The doctor and nurses ran over and thanked us; everyone was so happy that Mary was talking again.

Gunther, a twenty-five year old man, paralyzed from his neck down and unable to talk, can only respond with a smile and the blinking of his eyes. He enjoys our visits with the biggest smiles and the widest eye blinks.

Virginia sat in her room day in and day out, leaving only for a shower. She refused to join in any of the activities. However, when we visited, it was a different story. When she saw us walking down the hall, she called us into her room. Virginia is alert but disoriented to person, place and time. The interaction between her and the collies was just great. She carried on a conversation and reached out and stroked the dogs. When we left she asked us to please come back and visit with her again.

As a result of the work and volunteering that the dogs and I have done, we have won a number of awards and have been lucky enough to have stories written about us in several newspapers. I'm very proud of my dogs. We usually can get through to someone who hasn't reacted in a long time. I plan to continue volunteering my time with my best four-legged friends at all these homes and hope to inspire others to try it. I hope that if the time ever comes that I have to be in one of these homes, a program like this will be around for me.

I just want to thank Bubba for everything. I know she's up there, looking down on us. If it weren't for her, my three collies and I wouldn't be doing what we're doing today.

Guidelines As Set Forth By Therapy Dogs Inc.

1. Dogs must be at least one year of age to be eligible for registration with Therapy Dogs Inc.
2. Dogs must have all vaccinations current, including rabies, DHLPP and Corona-Virus.
3. Dogs must have an annual physical examination and stool check.
4. Handlers are encouraged to give participating dogs an annual heartworm test, dependent upon the area in which the dog will be working.
5. Female dogs must not be "in season" when participating in therapy visits.
6. Dogs must be well-groomed, clean and parasite-free; handlers must be well-groomed as well.
7. Dogs must be evaluated by a trained observer. This observer must complete the appropriate section on the registration form.
8. Dogs must be kept on a leash at all times when in an institution, except when doing certain obedience or trick demonstrations. Handlers are encouraged to use 4-foot leashes while participating in therapy visits. Large dogs may utilize a traffic lead.
9. Dogs must wear the red heart-shaped Therapy Dogs Inc. identification tag while participating in visits.
10. Rules and regulations in each facility visited must be followed strictly by all therapy dogs and their handlers. If these rules are unclear, the Chapter Coordinator/Director is obligated to consult an employee of the facility and to become familiar with these rules.
11. Basic training shall consist of knowledge including "sit," "down," "stay," "heel" and "come," performed reliably in the presence of extreme distraction.
12. It is advised that dogs be accustomed to working on a variety of surfaces, including grass, dirt, asphalt, carpeting and linoleum flooring. It is also helpful to have the dog become at ease while riding in elevators.
13. Dogs must prove to be well-socialized with other animals and people.
14. Caution must be taken when visiting frail residents in any institution. Bones may be brittle, skin may be easily torn or injuries may be aggravated by an overly enthusiastic dog or handler. Handlers must be aware that not every resident or attendee may wish

to make contact with their dog. Consideration of a variety of tastes must be taken into account while visiting.

15. At no time is a dog allowed to jump up onto the bed of any resident in a facility unless express permission has been given by an employee of the institution. This is for the safety of both the resident and the dog.

16. If any incident occurs while in an institution visiting under the name of Therapy Dogs Inc. that causes injury to an employee or resident or attendee in the institution, handlers must immediately contact their Chapter Coordinator/Director or the main Therapy Dogs Inc. office.

17. Dogs should be accompanied by a certified handler or trained observer for three (3) consecutive visits in order to assess the appropriateness of registration with Therapy Dogs Inc.

18. At the discretion of the Chapter Coordinator/Director, a handler and/or dog may be asked to temporarily or permanently refrain from further visits under the name of Therapy Dogs Inc. if the above guidelines fail to be strictly adhered to. Should this action be necessary, the handler shall immediately relinquish ownership of the red heart-shaped identification tags to the Chapter Coordinator/Director or directly to the main office of Therapy Dogs Inc.

For further information contact:

Therapy Dogs Inc.
Ann Butrick
PO Box 2786
Cheyenne, WY 82003
Phone: 307-638-3223

Behavior and Training

The Importance of Training
Brandy Lane Dog Training School

We have yet to meet a dog who could not be taught proper obedience. But only through proper education can the dog be made to clearly understand his proper place within your pack. The job of educating him — of making him understand his place — is up to you.

A dog can only be as good as the person who handles him and it is impossible for an uninformed trainer to obtain the same results as a trainer who is supplied with the facts. Once you have the knowledge, then you must depend on your desire, persistence, discipline and talent to produce the final results. The key to our method of training is that a dog is a dog. A dog is not an intellectual student who uses human logic. He is an animal who lives in a world without human logic. Learning is not accomplished through logical thinking, but solely through the faculty of memory presented through the medium of canine — not human — psychology. Attributing human characteristics to non-human creatures is called anthropomorphism. And while anthropomorphism might have a place in movies and fairy tales, it definitely has no place in dog training.

People who make the mistake of thinking that dogs are endowed with human understanding and morals never can attain a real relationship with their dogs. Our approach results in a happier, healthier dog, as well as a genuine relationship. The animal will not be required to master any command that exceeds his powers of comprehension. The trainer will avoid disappointment and annoyance because he or she will clearly understand the dog's abilities and will, hopefully, be able to attain real communication with the animal.

Becoming A Good Pack Leader To Your Dog

Before starting to teach any dog, the teacher should be familiar with how a dog thinks.

In its natural habitat, the wild, the dog belongs to a pack. If he is not the pack leader, he fits somewhere within the hierarchy (pecking order) of the pack. If he does not obey the laws of the pack, the leader will make certain that he complies. If the leader is not successful, a new pack leader will rise to take his place.

When you take a dog into your home, as far as he is concerned, he belongs to a pack. No dog ever turns on his master. Instead, he challenges for pack leadership. Therefore, if you are to be the pack leader, you must have a way of maintaining control over your dog. You must be able to establish definite rules and regulations from which the dog as a pack member can never deviate. And you must be in control at all times. If you are successful in enforcing your rules 99% of the time you are not the genuine pack leader. The 99% control will slip to 95% and then to 90% and eventually, if the dog has the drive toward achieving pack leadership, he might challenge. Fortunately for most people, most dogs prefer to remain as pack members and won't challenge for leadership.

You cannot gain 100% control over your dog if you employ such methods as hitting, kicking or in some other way abusing your animal. The dog will only come to mistrust those who strike him and will eventually bite out of fear or to protect himself.

Your dog will not automatically "pick up" your rules and regulations. He will have to be taught — and taught continuously — until he learns the proper behavior. But you must do your part as well. You must know what your rules are and then communicate them to your dog. This seems like an obvious point but you would be surprised at how many dog owners haven't taken the time to think out what it is that they want and expect from their dog.

Don't get the idea that this is going to be a life and death struggle for leadership between you and your dog. Actually your dog wants and needs a strong leader. Once he understands your rules and begins to obey them, he will be a much happier animal. So, for the benefit of your dog, it is up to you to educate him in such a way that he feels comfortable with your leadership. If you are unwilling or unable to do this, you really shouldn't own a dog in the first place.

Once the dog understands clearly what you want from him, he will respond in the hope of gaining your approval. This does not mean that your three-year-old or eight-year-old child will have the same control that you do. As far as the dog is concerned, he has one pack leader. The others in the family are pack members, each possessing position within the family hierarchy. He may adore your three-year-old but certainly won't obey him as he would the pack leader. The dog will obey each family member in direct proportion to that member's standing in the pack. One family member may get 90% control, whereas another might get 95%.

Maintaining Pack Leadership:

You should never ask a dog to do something unless you really want him to do it — but after you ask for it, you'd better make certain that he performs! Having your orders obeyed is a basic requirement in maintaining leadership. Naturally, while teaching a new concept, you can't get what you ask for immediately; however, once learning has been completed, then enforcement is necessary. This doesn't mean that you have to be cruel. On the contrary, you must be strong and yet offer love at the same time. The better you are able to combine these ingredients, the better a pack leader you will be.

It is important to understand that a pack hierarchy does not mean that the leader and the higher members will mistreat or abuse those below them. This is particularly important in families with children. If a youngster continually engages in ear-pulling, eye-gouging or tail-pulling, the dog will eventually come to mistrust the youngster. Therefore, the family pack members as well as the pack leader should be educated on how to treat the dog just as the dog must be taught how to live within the pack.

The dog should never be left unsupervised with a pack member who is not capable of physical control. The dog might play with this pack member as he would another dog — and this play can be rough and might result in physical injury to the youngster. If the dog is to be left free, there should always be some pack members present who are capable of assuming pack leadership. Some young children are capable of assuming this role with dogs; with other dogs, not even the man of the house is capable. Dogs and people are individuals; some people are stronger-willed than others and some dogs have stronger drives to be pack leaders.

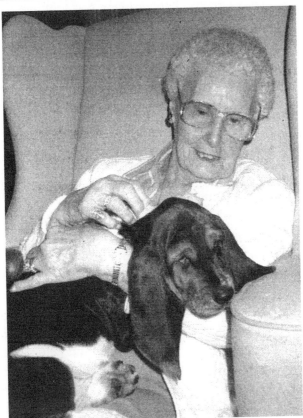

Ruth Elwood gives Lady Sadie "B" Good a welcome scratch as Lady visits residents in the facility.

Every Dog Needs a Number
by Charlotte Schwartz

Once upon a time, there were two dogs, a Cocker Spaniel and a German Shepherd Dog, who lived next door to each other. In each of the dog's houses there also lived a man, a woman and two teenage children.

One day the dogs were talking to each other over the fence in the backyard. The German Shepherd Dog was looking very glum that day and the Cocker Spaniel asked what was wrong.

"Oh, I don't know. I just can't figure out my pack. One day the man lets me sleep on his bed and tells me how handsome I look lying there with my head on his pillow. The very next day, when I lie on his bed, he comes into the bedroom and screams his head off at me. The next thing I know, he grabs me and when I growl at him, he thrashes me. Yet sometimes, I growl at the woman and she just leaves me alone — says I'm becoming mean. I'm confused," lamented the German Shepherd Dog. "Do you ever get confused in your house?" he asked his friend.

"My goodness, no!" said the Spaniel. "What's your number anyway?"

"What do you mean, what's my number?" asked the Shepherd.

"You know, your number. For example, my man is Number One, the woman is Number Two, their children are Numbers Three and Four and I'M NUMBER FIVE," explained the Spaniel, emphasizing the Number Five. "Isn't that great? It's wonderful to be Number Five!" she added, puffing herself up with pride.

The German Shepherd looked at his small, blonde friend and envied her such an important position in her pack. He wished he had a number and could be just as proud as she. But instead, he lowered his head and mumbled ever so softly, "I don't have a number. Nobody ever gave me one. How did you get yours?"

"Oh, I've always had Number Five, ever since I came here. I hardly remember how they gave it to me, but every once in awhile, when I get too excited or noisy or whenever one of my pack thinks

I'm being naughty, they remind me of my number. Then they always tell me how wonderful I am to be Number Five."

The little Spaniel lowered her sultry eyelids, wiggled her whole bottom and, with a self-assured twitch of her stubby tail, she pranced back toward her house. As she left, she said, "I hope you get a number someday."

With that, the handsome Shepherd went over to lie in the shade of a big maple tree and think about the conversation he'd just had with his friend next door. He wished he could talk so he could ask his family pack for a special number, too.

****

This little vignette is, of course, fiction, but the message it portrays is a proven fact. Pack animals such as dogs (and man) can only exist and flourish in a social group which has clearly defined hierarchy. And without the harmony which a hierarchy creates, the species cannot hope to perpetuate. In other words, the structure of an order of dominance in any social group insures its survival.

In the example above, the Cocker Spaniel will live out her life in peace and fulfillment, providing she continues to accept her number and is content with it. To her it is not important that she is Number Five; it only matters that she has a number. The only exception to this would be if she were unfortunate enough to live in a household where the humans made her Number One. In that case, she would fail because she would be incapable of making decisions and being responsible for the welfare of a pack of humans.

The case of her friend, the German Shepherd Dog, is another matter, however. Apparently, the social structure of his household is rather loose. Sometimes he's Number One in the hierarchy, sometimes he's Number Five and I'd bet money that there are also times when he fits somewhere in between.

The fact that he's allowed to lay on his master's bed doesn't necessarily mean he's Number One. Nor does the fact that his master removes him from the bed make him Number Five. But when he growls at his mistress and she walks away from him, he *thinks* he's dominant over her. That's the crux of the problem. And it creates a very dangerous situation for his entire pack.

When any individual in a social group does not clearly understand and accept a specific place in that society, it can mean trouble. And this "learning one's place" occurs in dogs as early as 12 to 16 weeks of age.

A litter of puppies, for example, begins to interact with each other by the time they are 21 days old. By three months, the puppies have developed a strong tendency to dominate each other. They bite, chew, growl, pounce and playfight. Through playfighting each puppy learns who it can dominate and who it must submit to. There is rarely bloodshed and severe injury, but there is a lot of ritualized behavior as each puppy learns to inhibit its aggressive tendencies and get along with its peers. Frequently, the largest and heaviest dog becomes the leader, Number One, and the others take up positions beneath him.

When a puppy goes to a new home, it needs to re-establish its position in the new pack. It's at this time in the puppy's life that knowledgeable owners help the puppy to make a smooth transition by showing it where it fits in the order of dominance in the new pack. In other words, it needs to be assigned a number.

Without the opportunity to interact with its own species when it is very young (before 16 weeks of age) and with man as it gets older (from 7 to 20 weeks of age), the puppy may grow up to be hyper-aggressive. A puppy who has been denied the opportunity to learn about social order at an early age finds accepting a position in any hierarchy later in life difficult if not impossible. These findings have been proven by many scientists and behaviorists over the last 40 or so years.

Finally, when a puppy enters the developmental stage of sexual maturity, he usually exhibits a resurgence of social dominance. In short, he attempts once more to climb the hierarchy ladder and dominate all those in his pack. If the owners are not aware of this behavior and the reasons for it, the dog can reach the top or leadership level, with disastrous consequences.

For example, an overindulged dog may assume a dominant role in the household. And the dog which is confused about its position in the hierarchy — one day he's "top dog" and the next he's "low man on the totem pole" — will become frustrated. Then the owners must deal with another problem, that of frustration-aggression.

However, knowledgeable dog owners are not only aware of the sexual maturity stage in the dog's life, but they know how to handle him so the dog will remain in his rightful position. Providing the dog is a normal individual and the maturity development stage proceeds without complications, the dog will remain a stable member of the social pack in which he lives.

How can a person tell, short of being bitten, if a dog is acting in a submissive or dominant manner? In his book, **Understanding Your Dog**, Dr. Michael W. Fox (1992) presents a list of behaviors which indicates dominance and submission by dogs. Here are some of the most common behaviors:

Dominant Behaviors:
- Stalking
- Growling, snapping, biting
- Baring teeth to reveal incisors and canine teeth
- Assumes "T" position with head over submissive dog's neck
- Pushing with shoulder or hip
- Walks around dog, stiff-legged, head and tail held erect
- Stands on subject's back
- Pushes dog down and stands over submissive dog

Submissive Behaviors:
- Lowers front part of body, tail tucked under
- Allows dominant dog to place feet on its back
- Retracts lips horizontally — raises forepaw
- Licks face area of dominant individual
- Tail between legs, ears back, directs gaze away from dominant dog
- Rolls onto back, remains still

- Urinates, defecates
- Sits or lies down and flexes one hip to expose inguinal (groin) area

These behaviors are ways in which dogs, using their bodies, speak to each other. We call it "body language." And for dog owners to live in harmony with canines, we should become familiar with and learn to use it.

The best example of this Dominance-Submissive sequence can be found between a dam and her puppies. Whenever a puppy behaves in a manner which is unacceptable to her (for instance, the puppy wanders away from the nest), she will go over to him, put her mouth over his head and her paw on his back. When he's down and possibly screaming as though he were being murdered, he will eventually relax under her paw. When the puppy no longer resists, the dam will remove her paw and walk away, sometimes eliciting a period of play from him.

Once an owner understands that his own body language speaks more clearly to his dog than any verbal language (dogs aren't born knowing how to understand words), then the owner can let the dog know he loves him, will assume responsibility for his welfare (dogs want a leader) and what position the dog must assume in the owner's pack. (Remember, man brought canines into his domicile — dogs did not bring man into their dens!)

It seems only common sense, then, to use one of the behaviors from the Dominance List to communicate to the dog that his place is beneath that of all the humans in the household. Doing that will achieve two objectives. It will let the dog know who is boss and it will give the dog a number of his own. (Remember the unfortunate German Shepherd Dog that didn't have a number?)

Making the dog lay down on its side, with its head and hips touching the floor, is an ideal way of communicating to the dog what his position is in the pack. We call this exercise the "Dominance Down."

The easiest way to accomplish a "Dominance Down" is to get down on your knees. Have the dog stand sideways in front of you.

Place both your arms over the dog's back. Now, take your two hands and reach over and through the center of the dog's body so that you can take his *inside* front leg in one hand and his *inside* back leg in the other hand.

Grasping both front and rear legs (the ones next to your body), firmly, but gently, pull the dog close to you and slide him down the front of your thighs until he comes to rest on the floor in front of you with his legs facing away from your body.

Next, take the hand that was holding his front leg and place it over his neck. The hand that was holding the rear leg now rests over his top or outermost, hip. Slowly stroke the groin area inside the top hip and you'll feel him begin to relax. The dog may even lift his topmost leg which is a further sign of submission to you.

It is important when placing the dog on his side to manipulate him smoothly and firmly. Do not slam or throw the dog down — you could hurt him. Do not be hesitant when you begin — this gives the dog time to resist you. Simply grasp his legs and, in one fluid motion, lower him to the prone position in front of you. Use your upper thighs as a slide to ease the dog to the floor — gravity will lower him down.

Now let's go back to Dr. Fox's list. This time we will study the signs of submission and look for one or more of them in your dog. He may lift his upper rear leg or attempt to roll on his back. He may even urinate. Whatever sign he gives you, he's saying, "OK friend. You're the boss!"

Occasionally, a person will own a dog which is naturally very submissive. He may or may not be aware of this. If you do a "Dominance Down" with just such a dog, you will notice almost immediately how submissive the dog really is to you. In this case, it is usually wise and not necessary to repeat it or it may make the dog even more submissive.

The very dominant individual will most likely resist you. The more a dog resists the "Dominance Down," the more determined he is to be the boss. This is, of course, the individual who most needs this exercise because man cannot live harmoniously with a dog which dominates him and all the other humans in a household. We simply cannot tolerate a dog running a human pack!

If the dog fights the "Dominance Down" by squirming, kicking, even screaming, you must react the same way his mother did. Growl at him. Don't yell "No! Stop that!" or "Lay down!" He won't understand and, furthermore, the panic in your voice will surely tell him he's getting the upper hand.

If you growl with a deep, emphatic voice, he'll get the message. Continue to hold him down with whatever force is necessary and show him (don't tell him!) that you mean what your body is saying.

Just as the puppy responded to his mother's "Dominance Down," your dog will eventually cease his resistance. You'll feel his whole body begin to relax under your hands. When you do, let him lay there for 20 to 30 minutes without moving and without your hands touching him. If he falls asleep, do not waken him until the time is up.

When you do, tell him, "OK, good dog!" and let him get up. Once he's on his feet celebrate with him, praise him, love him up all the while telling him how wonderful he is. Praise so enthusiastically that he gives you some form of recognition, a lick, a paw, tail wagging. Some behavior which tells you, "I love you and I'm not mad because you made me submit to you."

If you've done it correctly the dog will not only show you signs of affection, but he'll be more attentive, even more willing and eager to be with you. And you'll have opened a door to a deeper, more meaningful relationship with your dog.

For the next week, continue to do the "Dominance Down" every day for 20 to 30 minutes. A dog that is still fighting the exercise at the end of the week should continue for an additional week or whatever time it takes to make him understand. Eventually, however, even the most obstinate individual will give in and accept your leadership through the "Dominance Down."

One thing to keep in mind when you begin this program of establishing your leadership is that if you are working with an adult dog which has either been unsure of his position due to a lack of consistency on your part or one which has simply never been shown his correct position in the hierarchy, you will probably find it difficult at first. Occasionally, I've seen older dogs who had been overindulged all their lives and never came to accept a lower position in the pack.

In addition to the initial one week period of the "Dominance Down" exercise, the dog should be made to assume this position whenever his behavior is unacceptable to you. For example, if the dog barks incessantly at the arrival of guests and won't quiet down after you've admitted your friends (and he sees they're friendly people — not uninvited strangers), you can regain control very quickly by putting him in a "Dominance Down" for a minute or two.

If there are children in the home and dinner hour becomes somewhat chaotic as the kids and dog race around the house, have the children sit quietly with a book (yes, a quiet "down" with the children works wonders, too!). Next, put the dog into a "Dominance Down." Within minutes, you'll regain peace and order in the house. In other words, the "Dominance Down" simply says, "Hey, get a hold of yourself and watch your manners!"

By introducing the "Dominance Down" to any dog, you'll be giving the dog the most treasured gift a dog can receive. You'll be giving him a number that both of you can live with all his life. Remember, the dog doesn't care what position he has in the pack, providing it isn't Number One; it only matters that every dog needs a number.

Dog Crates — Cruelty or Kindness?
by Nicki Meyer, *Dog Fancy Magazine,* May 1984

Despite an almost universally negative first reaction, dog owners have come to swear by dog crates.

"He was such a cute puppy. If only he could have been broken of his bad habits. I really hated to give him up, but I just couldn't cope with it anymore. Perhaps someone else will have more time and patience."

These are familiar words to animal shelter workers. They hear them every day from frustrated owners who are "getting rid of" pets because of some sort of problem behavior. These workers are also aware that someone else probably won't have the patience and that, no matter how well-bred, attractive or appealing the dog may be, it will probably never find a permanent home or family and will soon become merely another euthanasia statistic. How ironic it is that, had the use of a dog crate been suggested to those same, well-meaning owners, their reactions would undoubtedly have been, "Put *my* dog in a cage? Never! It's a jail. It's cruel. He'd surely hate me. How could anyone be so mean?"

Is a dog crate cruel — or could it really be kind?

Perhaps the greatest mistake we devoted pet owners make is that we tend to consider our dogs "furry children." We fail to acknowledge and understand their mental limitations and strong animal instincts which persist despite centuries of domestication. We look at things from our viewpoint, not theirs. We expect, and often demand, more than they can deliver. It just doesn't occur to us to "think like a dog." If it did, there would be many more happy endings — and fewer animal shelters.

A puppy has many difficult adjustments to make when it enters its new home. Because it finds the world of humans confusing and perhaps frightening, it welcomes structure, routine, direction and control. Like its wild ancestors and relatives, it instinctively looks for a "pack leader" and seeks the comfort and safety of a "den." Of course it will deposit its waste anywhere and use its teeth on whatever is handy if it can, but it doesn't have to. Even young puppies are quite capable of bowel control and most will happily accept a substitute for the dining room furniture. Puppies want and need to please you. They do not choose to cause trouble and make you angry, but they often can't help it. Too much unsupervised freedom, which puppies can't handle, can quickly result in the development of problem behaviors that are difficult, if not impossible, to break. The proper use of a dog crate can start things off right — and keep them that way.

A dog crate may be a "cage" to you, but to your dog, it's simply a bed with a door or an indoor doghouse. The limited space and the fact that the door may be closed bothers you, not the dog. A young puppy not only accepts this type of confinement quite readily as a way of life, but also welcomes its security. Because it instinctively wants its den kept clean, the young dog rapidly learns to control its bowels itself, which makes for easier housebreaking. Since it naps frequently, it loves its cozy bed and it certainly deserves a private retreat where it can escape from active children or other types of stress. (Although the dog should learn to accept your reaching into the crate at any time, family members should respect a crate as a "special room" where the dog can go to be alone.) Above all, it needs to feel reassured when separated from its human "pack," both when left alone and when it must be restricted for convenience (family mealtime, guests, etc.).

An older dog has similar needs, which can also be met by a crate, though its adjustment to one may require some pleasant, positive conditioning and reinforcement. A crate can offer just the security a "problem" dog has been missing (which in itself could have triggered the behavior) and it can certainly help an adoptee adjust to a new home. In fact, far fewer adoptees would be available had they been given the benefit of a crate in the first place.

Most problem behavior, especially soiling and chewing, occurs when a dog, left entirely to itself in too large an area, becomes anxious, frustrated, bored or just plain lonely. Your negative reaction upon discovering the mess only makes things worse. Because it wasn't corrected in the act of misbehaving, the dog simply does not understand your anger and/or punishment, though the fear of it will certainly cause the dog to act "guilty." This results in even greater insecurity and often causes continued or even increased unacceptable behavior. It's truly a vicious cycle.

The greatest single asset of a dog crate is its effective control of a dog, especially a puppy, when it is left at home alone. The benefit to you, of course, is the peace of mind you enjoy when you are away from the house. Because your return is then a positive, not a negative, experience for both of you, the relationship you both desire can develop and grow all that much sooner. You are really doing your pet a big favor by keeping it out of trouble when it's left alone. Cruelty … or kindness?

Of course, a crate must be used properly and humanely. Its convenience should never be abused. It must be large enough to allow the fully grown dog to stretch out, sit up and turn around comfortably. (An adult crate can be blocked off for a puppy and the space enlarged as it grows.) It should be placed in a semi-private location — a corner is good — away from drafts or direct heat, but near enough to the household's center of activity so that the dog still feels very much a member of the family. It should contain proper bedding, toys and so on (but not water *unless* you are leaving the dog crated for more than an hour or two on a hot day; in which case the dog *must* have access to water. One solution is to invest in a water bowl which hooks onto the side of the crate.) It may be draped with a sheet or towel for added "den" coziness. It is after all, the dog's "own room." A puppy may be crated for up to four hours at a time and also at night once it has learned some bowel control; an older dog can go for up to six hours and at night. The crate was never intended, nor should it be used, for regular or frequent long-term confinement — all day, every day. Most dogs can be successfully and happily crated, though some may require firmness, conditioning and "convincing" before settling in. (There are, naturally, exceptions. Some dogs cannot or will not tolerate this form of restriction and react to it with hyper-anxiety, hysteria and/or violent behavior. In these rare cases, some other form of control is obviously indicated.)

The most practical type of crate for the pet owner is the collapsible one made of wire, though the molded fiberglass/plastic models are also popular. Its easy portability also makes the crate useful for travel or visiting, since the dog can ride safely in a station wagon, hatchback or van and always has its "security blanket" to help it feel at home in any strange surroundings. To be sure, not all crates compliment all decor's and they can be inconvenient and awkward if household space is at all limited. A crate can also be fairly expensive if the opportunity to rent one on a trial basis is not available. However, when you stop to consider its overall value to the dog and compare its cost to that of repairing or replacing furniture, carpeting, wallpaper or woodwork, it quickly becomes a real bargain.

For those opposed to its continued presence, it may not have to be a permanent fixture; once a young dog's good behavior is established and reliable, complete freedom may become entirely possible. Although the dog may miss the closeness and comfort it felt for the crate, it will probably remain trouble-free without it.

In a recent survey of dog owners, several hundred first-time users were asked to describe and evaluate their experiences with crates. Although the majority of respondents freely admitted to initially negative perceptions and reluctance to crating their dogs, their later testimonials were typically supportive and enthusiastic. "I don't believe it, he loves his crate." "I certainly wish I had know about them earlier. I'd never raise another dog without a crate." "It saved my sanity. We could never have kept the dog otherwise." "It makes traveling with the dog a delight and now we take him with us whenever we can." "Thanks to the crate, our puppy is always a pleasure and never a problem." "It's worth its weight in gold!"

Your dog desires little more in life than to please you. You, naturally, want to enjoy your pet and be pleased with its behavior.

Every dog deserves the chance to spend its life as the appreciated pet of a satisfied owner. A dog crate can truly help to make this relationship what each of you wants and needs it to be.

Two information-packed pamphlets are available to those who desire more information on crating. "Puppies, Parents and Kids," by Mordecai Segal, is available from the ALPO Center for Advanced Pet Study, PO Box 2187, Allentown, PA 18001. "A Pet Owner's Guide to the Dog Crate," by the author of this article, is available from the Nicki Meyer Educational Effort, 31 Davis Hill Rd., Weston, CT 06883. Enclose a stamped, self-addressed business-size envelope with each request.

Introducing Crate Training

Some dogs (especially puppies) take to crates immediately, or at least with very little effort on your part. Other dogs must be made comfortable with the idea over time. When introducing a dog to a crate, don't weaken and don't worry. Be firm and consistent and aware that you are doing your pet a favor.

For puppies, provide bedding in the form of an old towel or blanket (which can be washed) and some freshly-worn, unlaundered article of your clothing (tee shirt, old sweater, etc.). Avoid putting newspaper in or under the crate, since its odor may encourage elimination (corrugated cardboard is better if there is no floor pan). A puppy need not be fed in the crate and will only upset a bowl of water, though water bowls which hook on the side of a crate can be very useful. Whenever it is to be left alone for a while (remember, no more than four daytime hours at a stretch for pups), remove any collar and tags that could become caught and provide chew toys for distraction. If it is to be left in the crate on a hot day, it is vital that you *do* provide water for your dog or puppy.

A crate must be introduced gradually to an older dog, with every possible effort made to ensure that the dog's first association with it is positive and pleasant. Place the crate in a suitable location (see text, above), but do not put bedding inside yet. Prop the door open so that it cannot close suddenly and frighten the dog.

Encourage the dog to investigate thoroughly by tossing its favorite tidbits into the far end and praising the dog when it goes in after them and when it comes back out. Once the dog gains confidence, add whatever bedding the dog likes along with an article of clothing or a towel you have slept with. Next, encourage the dog to lie down and relax in the crate, still using food rewards if necessary. Continue this for several days, shutting the door briefly while you sit beside the crate. Do not hesitate to meet modest resistance with consistent firmness and authority so that the dog is clearly aware of the behavior you desire; your goal may have to be acceptance, not contentment.

Once the dog is accustomed to the crate (you may only be able to confine it for short periods at first), provide it with a safe chew toy when it's confined and be sure to remove its collar and tags.

Once again, use the crate sensibly. Properly used, a dog crate can make for a more confident, happier dog and fewer problem behaviors. However, long-term or frequent confinement at the whim of an often-absent owner can create as many problems as it cures.

Crate Manufacturers

As more people become aware of the benefits of dog crates, they will become more widely available. At present, however, crates are sometimes difficult to find in pet outlets. All of the following manufacturers produce quality dog crates. For more information on pricing and availability, contact these organizations:

- Anconco, 2221 Campbell, Kansas City, MO 64108.
- Central Metal Products, PO Box 396, Windfall, IN 46076.
- General Cage Corp., 238 North 29th St., Elwood, IN 46036.
- Kennel-Aire Mfg. Co., 731 Snelling Ave., St. Paul, MN 55104.
- Bob McKee Inc., 10864 Magnolia Blvd., N. Hollywood, CA 91601.
- Mid-West Metal Products, PO Box 2565, Muncie, IN 47305.

- Brandy Lane Dog Training School, 1162 King's Road, Mt. Holly, NJ 08060, Phone (609) 261-1321.

I Pity The Man
Author unknown

I pity the man who has never known
The pleasure of owning a pup;
Who never has watched his funny ways
In the Business of growing up.

I pity the man who enters his gate
Alone and unnoticed at night,
No dog to welcome him joyously home
With his frantic yelps of delight.

I pity the man who never receives,
In hours of bitterest woe,
Sympathy shown by a faithful dog
In a way only he seems to know.

I pity the man with a hatred of dogs;
He is missing from life something fine;
For the friendship between a man and his dog
Is a feeling almost divine.

Startup: Policies and Procedures for Dogs (and Puppies)

The following guidelines are taken from policies and procedures of The Masonic Home of New Jersey.

Guidelines For A Facility Dog

The following guidelines must be adhered to by all residents, staff and volunteers:

1. His name shall be (to be announced). Please do not use nicknames as they are confusing to an animal.
2. He is not allowed in any of the following areas:
    - eating or kitchen areas
    - bathroom areas
    - nurses stations
    - linen rooms
    - clean and dirty utility areas
    - laundry area
    - any storage areas
3. He shall always be either in his crate or on a leash.
4. Feeding: Please *do not* feed him any treats without Activity Staff permission. Treats, either special dog treats or table scraps, can lead to eating problems and obesity.
5. Picking him up: *Always* place one hand under his hindquarters and the other under his chest.
6. He will be trained with a "throw can." This is a simple home-made training device used to startle along with the word "*no*" to gain his immediate attention. This method will be used for all misbehavior and housekeeping mistakes.
7. Due to sanitation regulations, Food Service Employees will not be permitted to handle the puppy before or during their shift.

Masonic Home Puppy Schedule

7:00 a.m.: Picked up from Activity Room by resident, carried to outdoor location and allowed to urinate/defecate.

8:30 a.m.: Puppy is returned to the Activity Room for food and water. (He is allowed 15 minutes to eat, then the dish is removed; water is always available). Returned to crate.

10:00 a.m.: Picked up and carried outdoors for a short walk and visiting.

11:00 a.m.: Returned to crate.

12:30 p.m.: Feeding; picked up for outside walk and visiting.

2:00 p.m.: Returned to crate.

3:00 p.m.: Visiting in the medical center.

4:00 p.m.: Feeding, walking, visiting with responsible resident or returned to crate. He must be returned by 8:30 p.m. and the crate locked when the puppy is returned.

9:00 p.m.: Outside for nightly walk. Residents should return through door #2 and return the puppy to the crate and secure padlock. (The key should be picked up by the resident prior to 8:00 p.m. at the front reception desk.)

CRATE: The crate will be placed in the Activity Room at 8:00 a.m. by the Activity Staff and placed in the hallway at 4:00 p.m., except when an evening program is scheduled in Grow Memorial Hall. In that case it will be placed in the hallway after the program by the Activity Staff. A padlock will be placed on the door after the puppy is returned from the evening visit and again after his walk at 9:00 p.m.

Keys will be kept by:
1. the Activity Department
2. the telephone operator
3. the security department

My Puppy's Wish List

The following is only a *suggested* list. You may start with much less than I have suggested here, but this will give you a general idea of the items you might want to consider. If you have time to shop — perhaps a pet store in your area will give you a discount. I was fortunate enough to find someone who did. Every penny helps! However, if time is not something you have a lot of or, if your facility prefers, you can work through a purchase order system. I have included some catalog companies in the appendix that might be of help to you. Enjoy shopping. This is part of the fun of developing your program.

- **Folding Crate.** Folding crates are much easier than conventional crates to pick up and move about when necessary.
- **Imitation Lambs Wool.** This makes a great floor pad in the crate. Can be cut in smaller pieces for the puppy to make into piles and curl up with.
- **Bowls.** Bowls that hook on the side of the crate are great for uncoordinated pups. They help to avoid spilling or stepping in.
- **Water Holes.** These are special bowls to take on vet visits or whenever traveling — they keep the water from spilling.
- **Shampoo.** A must!
- **Grooming Tools.** These will vary depending on the type of pet you get.
- **Cleaners** for crate and spills etc. There are good cleaners available, however if your budget will not allow this, an ounce of bleach in a gallon of water will do the trick. Consult your housekeeping department also.
- A **Scooper** is a must. They have several names but all do the same job. Select one that is sturdy and will hold up for a long time. A good idea for traveling is a roll of paper towels and a box of large plastic bags; pick up the feces and discard in a local trash can.
- **ID Tags.** There is a difference of opinion with regard to what should be on the tags. Let this be your choice. It may include

the pet's name, your name and address and your phone number. At the very least include your last name and phone number.

- **Collars or harnesses and leashes.** A collar or harness is a must! They should have Rabies and License tags attached at all times.
- **Choke Chains.** *Never, never* have a choke chain on your pet except when walking or training. Remove as soon as the walking or training session is over. They can be dangerous and may be life threatening to your pet.
- **Toys.** An assortment of toys. Be careful of squeakers. Puppies like to chew them out of the toy and eat them. If you are lucky, they will pass them. If not, you may end up at the vets and possibly need them surgically removed!
- **Natural Bones.** These are great for play time in and out of the crate. Stuff the center with peanut butter, freeze them and give to the puppy when you want to occupy it for a while.
- **Rawhide Bones.** These seem to be a controversial item. I have heard that pieces can get stuck and cause problems in the digestive tract. This is probably a good question to ask your vet.
- **A Name.** (See the sample form below.)

Name The Puppy Contest

Our new puppy has arrived!!
Born *(date)* in *(city, state)* to *(father's name)* and *(mother's name)*.

Please submit your suggestions to *(person in charge)* by *(submission date)* before 9:00 A.M.

Name_____

Submitted by_____

Chapter 8

Cats

How To Select A Therapy Cat
by Pat Gonser, PhD, RN and Lori Kilburn, BS, RT

Dogs have long been recognized as "Service Animals" in assisting individuals who are handicapped. Examples of these service animals include seeing eye dogs, hearing dogs and wheelchair assistance dogs. Rarely have cats been recognized as assistance animals. Although cats have been found in Nursing Homes and Adult Day Care Centers as pets, interacting socially with residents, they have rarely been selected specifically for therapy. More often they are feral cats living in the area, rescued from animal shelters or dropped off by caring individuals. Although these animals can make effective social pets, guidelines need be established to assist health care providers in choosing appropriate cats for a therapy program.

Kintoi Cattery, in conjunction with Positively Unique Fur Friends (PUFF) and the Delta Society, is working on establishing criteria for the selection of therapy cats. The Delta Society's Pet Partners Program has established criteria that animal therapists must meet in order to participate in their program. Kintoi Cattery has bred Abyssinian, Somali and American Shorthair show cats for nine years and is currently breeding cats specifically selected for temperament and companionability. PUFF, established in 1991, currently uses three of their cats in their Animal Assisted Therapy Programs. In order to qualify as a PUFF therapy cat, a candidate must:

1. be at least one year of age before being selected for the program. This provides the facility with the knowledge that the cat has been effectively socialized, is friendly and is comfortable interacting with numerous people in a crowded setting. Additionally, a cat's immune system is more stabilized by this age. Older cats are less likely to become ill when exposed to various hospital borne microbes.
2. be fully inoculated. This includes routine inoculations as well as feline leukemia and rabies. This requirement insures that the cats are healthy.
3. be a participant in the Delta Society's Pet Partners Program. This includes passing a veterinarian's physical. Again, this guarantees the animal's health.
4. be temperament-tested using Delta Society Pet Partnership format. (See *Appendix*). This provides the therapist with the knowledge that the cat has been effectively tested and is known to be friendly in any and all situations.
5. be specifically home socialized to various situations including, if possible, dogs, other cats, crowds and frequency of handling. These activities guarantee that the animal and residents will interact effectively.

When PUFF begins a therapy program, the following format is followed:

1. An Animal Assisted Therapist (AAT) meets with an administrative member of the facility. The therapist is often accompanied by a therapy cat. At this time, general therapy goals are discussed, arrangements for therapy times are arranged and the type of group dynamics established.
2. After the program is established, the AAT meets with the program staff to assist in the selection of clients for the therapy group.
3. The program staff and AAT then meet with clients to assist in developing an individual therapeutic animal assisted therapy plan. Specific goals are set for each client at this time.

4. The AAT arranges with volunteers to provide a cat who best meets the criteria of a therapy situation. Sometimes the clients are best served by a cat and dog team. This can be arranged through PUFF.
5. Volunteers are apprised of the type of clients with whom they will be interacting. Some of our clients have severe Alzheimer's Disease while others have sensory deprivations. The specific disability determines the breed of cat needed.
6. After the therapy session is completed, volunteers and program staff evaluate the interactions. Each person contributes their observations and assessments of the sessions.
7. The program staff then notes clients' interaction on their health care record.

Currently, three cats are used by the PUFF program. Kintoi's I'M an MYO is a spayed Abyssinian. She is two years old and a retired show cat, earning the title Grand Premier in the Cat Fancier's Association. She was specifically selected for this program because of her winning personality and persistence in seeking attention. If clients fail to recognize her presence, she will bump their hands with her head and insist on being petted. MYO's size, five pounds, makes her ideal for a cuddle-up lap cat. She often settles down in a client's lap or on their chair table to wait for a pat.

The second feline used by PUFF is Sagacat's Surefire of Kintoi. She is a five year old Somali who is a Grand Champion. A Somali is a longhaired Abyssinian, which makes her an ideal therapy cat. She has all the playful qualities of the Abyssinian, with the added benefit of a thick plush coat. This is especially beneficial with clients who have sensory depravation. Surefire is extremely playful and assists clients with range of motion exercises. She is the only cat therapist PUFF uses who is not spayed, therefore she takes a few weeks off every year for maternity leave.

The final cat used in the program at the present time is Rexitune's Love Me Tender (Teddy). He is a neutered Cornish Rex who holds the title of Premier. A Cornish Rex has a Marcel wave coat that is very soft. Clients love to touch him, expecting a wiry texture. Instead, they are met with a rich soft coat. This again is excellent for touch therapy.

Currently PUFF uses only pedigreed retired show cats. An important rationale for this selection is that cats from specific breeds can be more efficiently temperament predicted. Some breeds are more interactive than others. Also, show cats must be amenable to handling. Our cats are handled from the day they are born. This attention assists the cat to be better prepared for work as an animal therapist.

The writers do not want to imply that shelter or rescued cats would not make good therapy cats; many of them may. We would, however, encourage those persons interested in working with these cats to work closely with the Delta Society. Their guidelines are beneficial in determining if a specific cat is qualified for a therapy program.

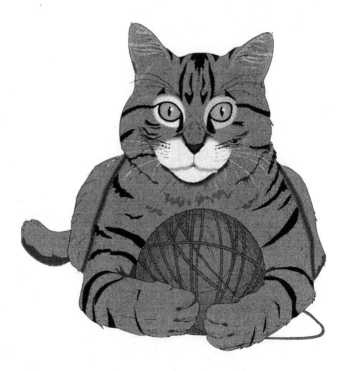

What A Difference A Cat Made!
by Lloyd A. Taylor, originally published in *Family Matters*

There she sat, all alone, waiting to be first in line for lunch. Every day at 11:30 she was just outside the door of the dining area. Only occasionally would any resident contest her place. Her name — Mrs. Saleeni; residents and workers called her "Sal" but never where she could hear them.

She was old, maybe 86, and walked with some difficulty, supporting herself with one crutch. She agreed with a 100-year-old resident just down the hallway who told everyone who would listen, "Its no fun to get old." What made it worse was that Sal was soured on life. Well, why shouldn't she be? Her husband had been dead so long she said she could hardly remember what he looked like. Theirs had been a childless marriage, so there was no one left to care. She had been very well educated for a woman of her day, but what good is a master's degree in English literature when your main concern in life is to be first in line for dinner?

She had lost her driver's license several years ago after a series of seven accidents in three months. She could no longer live safely in her little apartment; now she was a rest home resident. When she moved into the home, she had to abandon her eight beloved alley cats. No wonder Sal was soured on the world! She hardly ever smiled. She sat alone, for other residents could not abide her tart tongue. She continually intimidated the aides. Her self-imposed isolation intensified her feeling of aloneness which, in turn, made her even more caustic. What a vicious spiral she was in.

No one should have to live like this. I felt there surely must be some key to unlock this tightly closed personality and let a little joy come in. I tried speaking to her in the most friendly way I knew as I passed her each day. Her response was a scowl or some surly word muttered under her breath.

A nurse told me one day that they had to watch Mrs. Saleeni. She would take the meat from her plate in the dining hall and put it into the pocket of her blouse. When she got back to her room, she would open the little window and throw it to stray cats in the yard.

Sometimes, though, she would forget and the food would stay in her pockets for days. This casual conversation suggested that cats might be a way to reach Sal.

I have a cat. He is pure white and has only one front leg. Seven years ago, when he was a kitten dozing on a warm motor on a cold day, he lost one front leg in the fan belt pulley of my car. He is quite gentle for his leg was not all he lost when he was still a kitten. His name is P.K., short for Preacher's Kitty; he was the cat of the manse and terror of church mice before I retired.

One afternoon when P.K. had eaten himself into a state of lethargy I carried him to the home. Sal was still napping. When the nurse shook her awake she scowled and asked in a most negative way, "What do you want?" The nurse, not used to dealing with Sal's ability to wither people with words, said, "You have company," and fled.

Having a visitor was something new for Sal. She rolled over to see who we were. Instantly her scowl melted into a beautiful, though toothless, smile. When I put the cat on the bed he lazily stretched out beside her with his nose almost touching hers. She rubbed his head, scratched his neck and commented about his unusually long tail. Her smile never faded. P.K. and I stayed about 15 minutes. She was still smiling when we walked out.

What a difference a cat made. That day marked a drastic change in my relationship with Sal. She would spot me when I first walked into the home. She always smiled and spoke first. The administrator commented one day that I must be something special for she seldom spoke to anyone else. I told him that it was my cat that was special.

Each day she would ask, "How's the cat?" It was not long, however, before she rephrased the question, "How's MY cat?" A short time later she began asking, "How's my ANGEL cat?" That, of course, was a clear indication that she never owned P.K. for he certainly was no angel. I always have a funny story to tell her about the cat's antics. One day as I left her she told a lady standing nearby, "That man is taking care of my cat while I have to stay here." One day she told a nurse who was new on the floor, "That man takes such good care of my cat for me." The nurse saw me a little later and commented, "I think you are such a nice man to care for Sal's cat the way you do." Imagine her surprise to hear the full story.

Do you think I will ever tell Sal the truth about P.K.? Of course not! Why rob a lonely little lady of the one great satisfaction she has left? And what does P.K. think of the dual ownership? If he could comprehend, I am sure he would switch his tail in sheer glee and say, "You and Sal are both wrong. Don't you know, nobody ever really owns a cat?"

Startup: Policies and Procedures for Cats

The following guidelines are adapted from policies and procedures of The Masonic Home of New Jersey.

Guidelines For A Facility Cat

The following guidelines must be adhered to by all residents, staff and volunteers:

1. His name shall be (to be announced). Please do not use nicknames as they are confusing to an animal.
2. He is not allowed in any of the following areas:
   - eating or kitchen areas
   - bathroom areas
   - nurses stations
   - linen rooms
   - clean and dirty utility areas
   - laundry area
   - any storage areas
3. He shall always be within the building to avoid contact with wild animals and other sources of germs and parasites.
4. Feeding: Please *do not* feed him any treats without Activity Staff permission. Treats, either special cat treats or table scraps, can lead to eating problems and obesity.
5. Picking him up: *Always* pick him up carefully with two hands providing a much support as possible.
6. He shall always wear identification including the name and phone number of the facility.
7. A veterinary checkup including all required vaccinations will be made before he is brought into the facility.
8. Due to sanitation regulations, Food Service Employees will not be permitted to handle the cat before or during their shift.

Chapter 9

Rabbits

Rabbits can be a valuable addition to a pet therapy program. They are usually not quite as friendly as a dog or cat (depending upon the cat), but a quiet and gentle rabbit will be more appropriate for some residents. The right rabbit, living in the facility, will always provide an attraction for residents who are passing by.

The pluses: Besides being quiet and gentle, rabbits appreciate affection. They can be kept in a cage within the facility so they are always available to residents. Fewer people are allergic to rabbits than to some of the other furred pets. And they are "cute," which is an important aspect of why people like to have them around.

The minuses: Rabbits have a tendency to be frightened easily. Some rabbits "kick" hard enough to cause significant scratches (these rabbits clearly don't belong in a long term care facility). When a rabbit escapes, it can be very hard to find and catch. If rabbits are allowed to run free, they may chew on wires and other inappropriate items.

On the whole, though, a gentle rabbit which is accustomed to being around people adds another valuable dimension to a pet therapy program. As the following articles will demonstrate, they may be successfully used either as visitors or as facility pets.

The Floppy-Eared Therapist: A Message To Directors
by Sue Steganga, Sacramento, CA

One of the most effective and sensitive therapists I know of has gigantic ears and enormous feet, though he's really quite small in stature. Some folks think he's somewhat peculiar looking and he's certainly not a typical therapist. But most of his advocates think he's adorable in his own unique way. Not only does he have huge floppy ears and clodhopper feet, but he also has a nose that wiggles in excitement as he hops from place to place. You guessed it: this therapist is a rabbit — a Holland lop rabbit, to be exact.

His name is Bambi. I know, I know. Rabbits are supposed to be named Thumper. But ever since my childhood days, I've dreamed of adopting a pet deer and that never quite happened. And since my bunny is so gentle, tender-hearted and the color of a fawn, it seemed logical to me to name him Bambi.

I first considered adopting a rabbit after I accepted a new job and moved to a location far from my family and longtime friends. Because I am a single woman, I decided I needed a pet to greet me when I came home to my quiet apartment. Of course, animals are also considered wonderful companions and contribute to the good health of anyone who lives alone. Since I was gone all day and lived in a tiny studio apartment, I figured housing a dog was out of the question. I seem to have developed a slight allergy to cats. (My allergist tried to convince me to adopt something without fur such as a fish or a snake, but I couldn't imagine cuddling up to one of those critters.) Anyway, a rabbit sounded like a reasonable alternative to me because it could be in a cage while I was at work. Then I could let it out to play when I got home. So that is how I came to have a bunny as a "roommate."

Did I ever grow fond of this little guy! He was a real character with a lovable personality, yet he was also strong-willed and independent. Nevertheless, at first he became very shy around visitors. But I encouraged my new friends and their young children to come over to pet and play with him so he would become more relaxed around other people. Soon I discovered that friends of all ages were charmed by his humorous antics.

I eventually moved back to my hometown and my bunny moved along with me. A few years ago, an elderly friend from my church had a sudden stroke. I began visiting Retta in her assisted-living setting. Before her stroke, Retta had been a very active and articulate woman. It was extremely frustrating for her to struggle to communicate verbally after her stroke. When she could not recall a particular word in the midst of a conversation, she would become frustrated and apologize profusely. Much as I attempted to encourage a two-way conversation so she could continue practicing speaking, I often found myself rambling on in a monologue about any topic that came to mind. One day I happened to mention my bunny and his latest antics. Retta's face brightened. She smiled and giggled. I realized that I had discovered a topic that entertained and amused her. After that time, I talked often about my bunny and would send Retta greeting cards (especially at Easter) from my bunny.

It was difficult to watch Retta's physical decline during the next few years. She was eventually moved from an assisted-living situation to a more full-scale nursing home. I had read that rabbits have been utilized in therapy sessions for nursing home residents. So I asked permission from the home to bring in the rabbit for short visits. Retta loved seeing and petting Bambi, without feeling any pressure to speak. In fact the bunny's non-judgmental and accepting presence encouraged her to speak once in a while without being concerned about saying "the right words."

Retta had several more strokes and continued to fail physically, although she stayed mentally alert. I would stop by with my bunny for brief visits even when any conversation had become too difficult. But with an animal to cuddle, words were no longer important. My sensitive bunny seemed to understand the need to be particularly gentle around this special lady.

The time came when I knew that this would probably be my final visit with Retta. When I entered the room, Retta was in a deep sleep. I whispered her name and told her that I had brought the bunny to see her. Retta didn't stir or respond. I waited a while and was just about to leave. But something inside me seemed to tell me to hold the bunny near her to say good-bye. So I held the bunny close to Retta's cheek and rubbed his soft fur gently against it. I explained to her that what she felt was the bunny's fur. Retta never opened her eyes but I noticed that her lips quivered slightly. I think she was trying to acknowledge our presence. I couldn't bring myself to say "good-bye" and instead whispered, "see ya later, Retta." I took one more look at my dear elderly friend, Retta. Then I put my furry little friend, Bambi, back into his traveling cage and hurried out the door. When I got to my car, I just sat there clutching my bunny's cage. He looked at me inquisitively with his chocolate brown eyes, so I gently lifted him from his cage. I stroked his velvety soft fur and held him close as he licked the salty tears that trickled down my cheeks. Yes, my floppy-eared friend was excellent "therapy" that day — not just for my dying friend, but also for me as I sadly drove away.

Hints for Rabbit Visitations

Reprinted by permission of Gary Grimm and Associates
Copyright 1995 Gary Grimm and Associates
Publication "A New Day" March-April 1995

Rabbits have therapeutic value in full-care nursing homes and assisted living settings. They are distinctly different from other domestic pets and have their own special characteristics. Here are some hints for taking a rabbit to visit the elderly:

The rabbit should be old enough and comfortable being around unfamiliar people. It should also be accustomed to being held and housebroken. A young, nervous, and/or restless rabbit may squirm and wiggle, and may hop out of your arms.

Never bring in a rabbit that has shown abnormal or aggressive tendencies or has nipped, kicked or scratched anyone. Be aware that any animal may act differently in a new environment or when frightened. Remove a rabbit that acts strangely.

A rabbit raised by a reliable breeder and living in a loving home environment is generally more gentle and predictable than a rabbit from a pet store, where the rabbit may have been poked and prodded. Although a rabbit from a pet store may be accustomed to that kind of treatment from customers, as a result it may have developed an unfriendly disposition and distrust of strangers. If a rabbit *is* brought directly from a pet store for a visit, make sure the person who brings it in knows the rabbit's temperament and how to hold and handle it properly.

Generally, only the owner should hold the rabbit. The owner will probably need to hold the rabbit close to his or her body, which makes the rabbit feel secure and less likely to wiggle or hop away.

Rabbits must never be held by their ears. Wrapping the rabbit's lower body in a small baby blanket or towel makes it easier to hold the rabbit securely and makes it feel safe. The rabbit will look adorable with its little head and ears poking out.

Find out if anyone at the residential facility is highly allergic to animals and avoid exposing anyone to rabbit dander who might be endangered. Fortunately, people are less likely to be allergic to rabbit dander than that of more common pets, such as cats.

A rabbit will stay calmer if you bring it in to visit rooms with only one resident or a few people present at a time. The rabbit is less likely to be distracted in a small, quiet room. Rabbits become easily frightened by loud noises or sudden movements.

Encourage residents to speak softly when nearby and when talking directly to the rabbit. Remember that some people who are hard of hearing may speak more loudly than the rabbit is used to hearing.

If residents or staff want to pet the rabbit, hold the back of the rabbit towards them to be petted, with the rabbit's face away from them. This prevents someone from accidentally poking the rabbit's eyes or from scaring it by coming too quickly towards its face. Encourage petting on the back of its body rather than on the head.

Cradle the rabbit's head in your arms and guard its mouth so it can't nip anyone.

Do not let anyone feed the rabbit unplanned treats. Even vegetables such as carrots may make the rabbit ill if these tidbits are not part of the rabbit's regular diet. Only the owner should feed the rabbit.

Avoid putting the rabbit outside in direct sunlight for a long time, since rabbits can become overheated very easily. If you take flash photos of the rabbit with residents, hold the rabbit securely in case the flash of light startles it.

A rabbit makes a good subject for initiating conversations and stimulates memories about treasured pets. For instance, when I showed my bunny, many folks reminisced about rabbits that they had raised and other pets they missed, such as dogs and cats. Several of the residents thought it was a "nice kitty." And one gentleman laughed and suggested that I might want to keep the rabbit away from him because he used to hunt rabbits years ago!

Rabbit Therapy at the Baptist Home of South Jersey
by Harriet Ciccotosto

The most recent addition to the Baptist Home staff is "Funny," a five-month old gray dwarf rabbit, who requires much more in the way of care than the pet birds that were already here. She was donated to the facility by a friend of a staff member. Our veterinarian advised us that it would be necessary to concentrate on "socializing" Funny, as rabbits are not generally considered to be the social animals that cats and dogs are. This means providing daily contact with residents so that Funny will be "people friendly" — comfortable with their constant attention. Some aspects of our experience with this rabbit therapy program are described below.

Resident Involvement

Residents interact with Funny on a daily basis, either by coming to the Activity Room for a visit or through one-to-one visits in the residential and nursing care areas of the facility. These visits are supervised by Activity Professionals. The rabbit elicits positive reactions from a majority of residents through petting and/or observing her behavior.

Benefits to the Residents

Funny has contributed much to our Home, as well as providing a great topic for conversation.

The process of familiarizing Funny with the residents has elicited a nurturing response in many of the female residents. This is particularly true of those from the nursing care unit, who seem to want to protect and look after her at all times.

The tasks of cleaning the cage, changing the food and water daily and even buying the food, have provided incentive for the residents to become involved and attached to Funny. She serves as a "portable socialization tool" who draws attention wherever she goes.

Drawbacks to Keeping a Rabbit

Compliance with state and federal regulations make it necessary to keep animals away from areas where food and medicines are being dispensed. This means that Funny cannot be at liberty at any time. Also, Funny sometimes likes to nibble and chew on things that she shouldn't. This requires disciplining her, either by clapping loudly to signal disapproval or by giving her a light tap accompanied by saying a harsh "NO!"

There *are* minor drawbacks to keeping a rabbit at a facility, but they have been more than compensated for by the joy that these pets have brought to residents, staff and visitors. And Funny has proven to be an excellent addition to our program.

Policies And Procedures for Rabbits

Policy:

To provide for an in-home residence Pet Therapy program. The responsibility for the registration of all pets within the facility will be handled through the Activity Department. The health maintenance and care of the in-home rabbit and the logging of appropriate veterinary records will also be maintained by this department. In the event of the death of the rabbit, replacement costs will be deducted from the Activity Department operational budget.

Procedures:

1. The rabbit will be approved by the Administrator and/or the Board of Trustees of the facility.
2. The rabbit will be examined by a veterinarian to ensure freedom from disease, parasites, etc.
3. The rabbit will be kept in the Activity Office and cared for by the Activity Staff and resident volunteers as needed for weekends, holidays, etc.
4. The rabbit will be effectively controlled by a cage.
5. The cleaning of the cage and the purchasing of food and needed supplies will be the responsibility of the Activity Staff.
6. During Pet Therapy visitations with residents, an Activity Staff member will be responsible for the control of the rabbit.

Chapter 10

Birds

Bird Therapy at the Baptist Home of South Jersey
by Harriet Ciccotosto, SCC

Peter and Paul, our two in-home pet English parakeets, have been with us for about a year and a half now. They were purchased after an initial interest survey of residents (living in both the residential and nursing areas of the Home) revealed that a great need for in-home pets existed. Many of the residents had kept birds, fish, cats, dogs, etc. and missed the daily contact and enjoyment that these pets had provided in their lives.

The parakeets were purchased with funds taken from the Activity Department operational budget. With this money we bought two birds, a cage, a stand and start-up supplies. Everything were purchased at a discount from a local store that specializes in birds. (It was found, after researching prices, that it was more cost-effective to make our purchase in this specialized store.) Supplies needed to maintain the birds are also taken from the departmental budget.

As the birds are located in a communal area of the Home, residents are involved with them on a daily basis. Many will stop to visit or talk with Peter and Paul on their way through the halls or before or between activity programs. Several residents have volunteered to change their food and water and to assist with the cleaning of their cages.

In addition to stimulating conversation, the parakeets have added greatly to our Home. They have given a sense of purpose to two residents who have tended to be somewhat self-isolating and minimally active. The care and feeding of the birds has been a welcome responsibility for them. For another of our residents, who was the winner of our "Name Those Birds" contest, they have brought special meaning. They remind her of the birds she had in her younger years and she considers herself their adoptive "mother."

The birds provide visual and auditory stimulation which is much enjoyed by the residents who are more regressed. It is not uncommon to see some of them simply sitting beside the cage and observing Peter and Paul's actions.

One negative aspect of having birds is that they present additional work for the housekeeping department when they are molting. They can also be disruptive during some programs because they are kept in a heavily trafficked area where they can become easily excited. It was discovered that this problem could be overcome by covering the cage, which quiets them immediately.

Another problem that we've experienced with parakeets is that they tend to become lethargic when the weather becomes too warm or humid. This was easily solved by moving them from their normal area, where there is no air conditioning, to another where there is air conditioning twenty-four hours a day.

Residents also tend to feed Peter and Paul inappropriate "treats." A boldly printed sign reminding them not to feed the birds has been affixed to the cage.

The few minor drawbacks of keeping the birds have been greatly outweighed by the joy they have brought to residents, staff and visitors. They have proven to be a most welcome addition to our home.

Policies And Procedures for Birds

Policy:
>   To provide for an in-home resident pet therapy program. The responsibility for the registration of all pets within the Home will be handled through the Activity Department. The health maintenance and care of the in-home birds and the logging of appropriate veterinary records will also be maintained by this department. In the event of the death of one or both of the birds, replacement costs will be deducted from the Activity Department operational budget.

Procedures:
1. Birds will be approved by the Administrator and/or the Board of Trustees of the facility.
2. The birds will be examined by a veterinarian to ensure freedom from disease, parasites, etc.
3. The birds will be kept in an appropriate residential communal area and fed and cared for by the Activity Staff and resident volunteers.
4. The birds will be effectively controlled by a cage.
5. An alternate resident volunteer or staff member will be responsible for feeding the birds should the designated resident volunteer be unable to fulfill this responsibility.

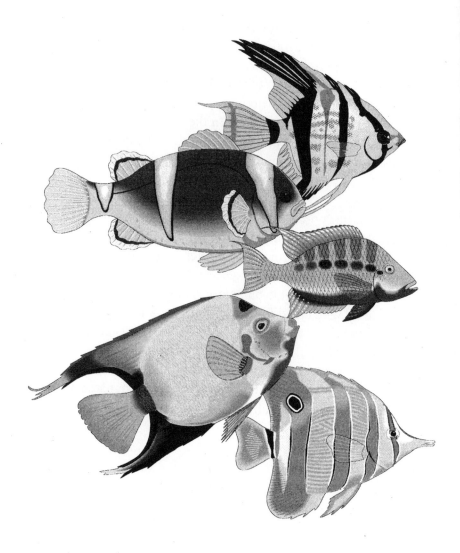

Chapter 11

Fish

Research on the use of fish in geriatric settings has produced mixed results. Not very many studies have shown significant physiological changes as a result of watching fish. (One study that showed positive changes was Cutler Riddick, 1985.) One study also shows that the residents report feeling more relaxed or less on edge after watching fish (Gowing, 1984). Other studies show no effect or small effects from watching fish.

On the other hand, no one has suggested that watching fish causes any harm to residents. Even in the studies which showed no significant effects, the researchers suggest that further studies, looking at different aspects of the problem are justified.

What does this mean for you if you are thinking about using fish as part of a therapy program? Fish are a pleasing addition to a facility but there are probably better ways to spend your money and time if your concern is for improving the condition of your residents. This is not to say that you shouldn't have a fish tank and, if residents request one, you should get one. We only want to suggest that the connection between a pet therapy program and getting a fish tank should not be automatic. The rest of the chapter shows the procedures used at the Masonic Home for their fish tanks.

Fish Tank Instructions

1. Only community fish will be placed in the fish tanks.
2. The fish will be fed with freeze-dried food which is to be kept in the work closets on each floor.
3. **Feeding** is done in the following manner: A pinch of food is dropped into the tank. If it is completely eaten by the fish, another pinch may be added until the fish have had enough to eat. The fish will be fed once daily, in the morning. The fish will be fed by Activity Staff or designated residents only. All others, please do not feed the fish. While fish can live for three months without food, they will be fed daily. While feeding the fish, turn the filter to the **negative** side to slow the filtering system. Return to the previous position when feeding is completed.
4. If a fish is found dead in the tank, remove it with the net found in the cabinet under the tank. Check to see if the fish has been attacked by another fish, then flush the dead fish down the toilet. If a fish has been mutilated in any way by other fish, stand back from the tank and try to find which of the other fish is the attacker. If the attacker is a large fish in a tank with smaller fish, it can be removed and put in a tank that has larger fish. If the dead fish appears to be completely intact, check the tank. If the tank is cloudy, remove 1/3 of the water and replace it with water from the tap that has sat out for 24 hours.
5. **Introduction of new fish:** Observe the size of the bag in which the fish has been delivered. Remove enough water so that the bag can be immersed into the tank. Float the bag in the tank for ten minutes, attaching it to the hood. Open the bag and add water from the tank to double the amount of water that was originally in the bag. After 10 minutes, remove the bag and let the fish swim in the tank.
6. **Thermometers:** Each tank has a thermometer. The temperature in the tanks should be maintained between the high 70's and low 80's.

7. **Heater:** to turn the heater on, remove the cap, tighten the knob to turn the heat on. Loosen the knob to lower the heat. The light on the thermometer in the tank will light when it is heating.

8. **Water** will be changed in the tank once per month. This will be done by removing one-third of it and replacing it with tap water that has sat at room temperature for at least 24 hours.

9. No cleaning fluids of any type will be used on the tank or on the hood. Warm water on a paper towel may be used to remove finger prints from the tank.

10. **Fish** will be replaced at two week intervals when needed.

11. **Lighting:** the tank light will be turned on in the morning and turned off in the evening at 4:00 p.m. If the light is turned on in the evening for residents, please be sure that its turned off by 11:00 p.m.

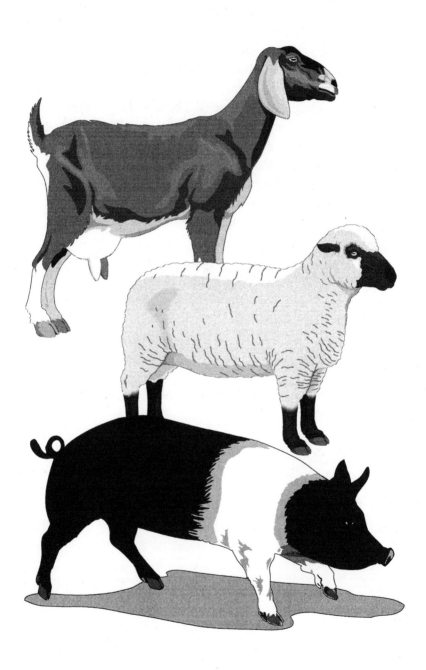

Chapter 12

Farm/Barnyard Animals

Potbellied Pigs

A more recent participant in the pet therapy arena is the "potbellied pig." These are happy, friendly and enthusiastic creatures. They seem to thrive on attention, are always willing to get dressed up for the occasion and often do tricks. They are clean and can be housebroken. Some are even trained to ring a bell that hangs on a door when they want to be let out for potty breaks.

A rather famous pig from New Jersey who made his TV debut on NBC's "Do Something," a broadcast that "features people who do something to help their fellow man" (*Animals Exotic and Small Magazine* — October 1995 by Alice Randall-Riley), created quite an "unexpected and remarkable transformation" in the facility where the taping was being done. It was reported that the taping increased socialization and self-esteem more than any other event that the staff had planned.

In recent years, potbellied pig associations and clubs have sprung up all over the United States. There are now two national organizations which serve the needs of those interested in any aspect of these animals, from breeding and raising, to healthcare and pet care (see *Appendix*).

The Delta Society now certifies pigs as "Pet Partners." Believe it! It happened to a black pig named Pumpkin. He was applying his charm for everyone on the day he passed his test. His owner, a speech pathologist, told the story of a client whom they could not encourage to speak until the day she took Pumpkin to the facility with her. The client has been speaking ever since.

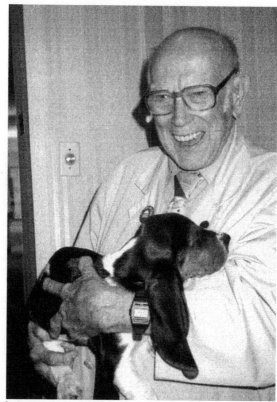

Earl Green's smile tells the story. Puppy love is a wonderful thing!

Chapter 13

Health and Safety

Transporting Pets

How Should A Therapy Pet Be Transported?

It is a great feeling to travel down the road with your wonderful dog along side of you; people wave and smile at the stoplights, some even roll down their windows and make nice comments. However for the safety of your pets, the number one choice for transporting them is in a crate. The crate should be large enough for your pet to be comfortable but should confine it enough so as not to allow it to be thrown if a sudden stop occurs. A second choice would be a pet seat belt. This fits around the dog's body. Then the seat belt of the vehicle fits through a loop in the pet belt to secure the pet on the seat.

These two methods could also be life saving for you. One of the trainers we worked with told us a story about a friend who had been in an auto accident. The man was seriously injured and needed medical attention. However, his dog, who was uninjured in the accident, would not allow anyone near the injured victim. Fortunately, the incident occurred just a few blocks from the victim's home. Someone summoned his wife and she was able to comfort the dog and remove him from the scene so that medical help could be given to her husband. Animals show great concern when they sense that you are ill or hurting. They will protect you from strangers. In a case like this their protective instincts could be life threatening to you. Using a crate can avoid this type of incident and provide your pet with the safety it needs.

How Can I Transport My Therapy Pet On Hot Days?

Simply, very carefully. If you transport your pet each day you may have to make adjustments in your regular routines. For example, my husband and I travel together in our van with our two dogs in their crates. On hot summer days we must take the dogs home first, then go back out and do the errands, etc.

The Humane Society of the United States gives the following information about pets left in cars in hot weather.

Leaving Your Pet in a Parked Car Can Be a Deadly Mistake

On a warm day, the temperature in a parked car can reach 160° in a matter of minutes, even with partially opened windows. With only hot air to breathe, your pet can quickly suffer brain damage or die from heatstroke.

Signs of heat stress: heavy panting, glazed eyes, rapid pulse, dizziness, vomiting, deep red or purple tongue.

If your pet gets overheated, you must lower his body temperature immediately! Get him into shade and apply cool (not cold) water all over his body. Apply ice packs or cold towels only to head, neck and chest. Let him drink small amounts of cool water or lick ice cubes or ice cream. Get your pet to a veterinarian right away — it could save his life.

On hot days, your pet is safer at home!

The Humane Society of the United States, 2100 L Street, NW Washington, DC 20037 (201) 452-1100.

Spaying/Neutering Issues

Should I Spay/Neuter My Therapy Pet?

This is a question you must think about carefully before making a decision. What will produce the healthiest and most desirable outcome for the pet? Most vets recommend spaying/neutering unless you want to show or breed your pet. Keep in mind that pets have rights! The figures drawn from statistics on this issue are staggering. More than ten million cats and dogs are euthanized annually. However, if you have obtained your pet from a breeder who particularly breeds for temperament and therapy work and your pet is an outstanding performer, the breeder may request to have a litter from it. You will then need to decide if this is something that you want. If your pet is a male who would provide stud service, you would only need to be sure to get pictures for your residents and possibly have a visit from the puppies — after their shots and just before leaving for their new homes. If you have a female, however, you would need to ask yourself some difficult questions:

- Could you and/or the residents handle her absence for eight weeks while she births and cares for her puppies?
- Would you consider allowing the pups or kittens to be born in the facility?
- Would you even have an appropriate area for a whelping box or be able to provide adequate care for the puppies?

If you're still enthusiastic — think again! I know some folks — staff and residents alike — who would love it if a litter were born to their therapy dog. Being an old obstetrical nurse myself, *I* would love it. But this scenario would probably only really work in one in a million facilities. Think about moving in with your sleeping bag for the entire 6-8 weeks. There are not too many residents or staff who could cover for this period. Think about the mother. What would happen if she becomes overwhelmed by more than she could handle; visitors in her area and people handling her pups during those hours when you could not be on hand? Rules are so often broken and it would be so tempting for folks to handle those precious little pups. Would you want to undo her as a therapy dog?

Another issue to consider might be fund raising — are you, as the Activity Director, required to do your own? Would the risks and time required justify the funding this provided to your department? This is something I would have to ponder long and hard.

One possible solution might be for a breeder to keep the dog when her due date is near and handle the birthing process and the first 6-8 weeks of the new puppies' lives. Even so, there is yet another factor to think about. Can you find homes for all the puppies? Remember those ten million cats and dogs that are euthanized each year! Animal welfare groups hold both the stud owner and the female owner equally responsible for the placement of the offspring.

In summary, spaying/neutering is probably the best choice for a therapy dog. For the female it eliminates the possibility of an unwanted pregnancy and the need to leave her at home during estrus. For the male, it eliminates unbecoming behavior while in the facility and decreases the risks of cancer. Some experts believe that neutering also leads to the development of a more "laid back" personality in the male.

Ticks

Are Ticks A Real Problem For Pets?

Yes! W. Bradford Swift, DVM stated in an article for *Dog Fancy Magazine*, August 1991: "A bite from this bloodsucking parasite can cause serious problems." The four most commonly known diseases that can be transmitted are

- Rocky Mountain Spotted Fever
- Lyme Disease
- Tularemia
- Tick Paralysis

An in-depth description of these diseases can be found in the above mentioned article. Dr. Swift notes that ticks are most common from May to August. However, some areas have ticks year round. His recommendations for prevention of Tick Borne Diseases include: wear long pants tucked inside socks, wear light color clothing to make visibility easier, keep grass cut short, use tick repellents, combine insecticide and repellents on your pets and lastly vaccinate your pets against Lyme Disease.

To remove ticks he recommends the following: Remove ticks carefully with a fine pair of tweezers. Grasp the tick as close to the head as possible. Exert gentle but steady pressure until the tick lets go. Immediately clean the area with soap and water. Try not to crush the tick with your fingers or with the tweezers. Kill the tick by dropping it into alcohol.

For more information on Tick Borne Diseases, see *Chapter 14, Infectious Diseases.*

Hip Problems

Will Large Dogs Develop Hip Problems?

Canine Hip Dysplasia (CHD) is a genetically transmitted disease that may not only affect the hip joint, but may also affect the "elbows, shoulders and even the joints between the vertebra." (May 1995, *Dog World*). This is a complex topic to summarize in a few short paragraphs. As an Activity Professional, you should be discussing this subject with the breeder. Also ask for copies of the litter's parents' Orthopedic Foundation of America rating. If they have good hips, chances are your pet will too. Yet, unexplained occurrences of CHD have happened. If you do find your dog has hip dysplasia, do not be alarmed. If you are not planning to breed and it is not severe, the pet will live a normal life, although there is the possibility of pain and discomfort occurring in later years.

For in-depth and understandable reading about this disease, please refer to *Dog World Magazine* starting with the May, 1995 issue — "Canine Hip Dysplasia Part I" by John C. Cargill, MA, MBA, MS and Susan Thorpe-Vargas, MS. Another interesting article is one on hip replacement. It can be found in *Second Opinions* — Veterinary Referral Associates, Inc., Fall 1994, 15021 Duties Mill Road, Gaithersburg, MD 20878 Phone: (301) 340-3224.

The following paper prepared by International Canine Genetics, Inc. will answer some questions you may have relative to Canine Hip Dysplasia and a new technique to discover it as early as 16 weeks of age. My special thanks to Dr. Stephen T. Peterson, DVM who so kindly allowed this paper to be printed in its entirety.

PennHIP: Questions and Answers about PennHIP

New Scientific Method for Early Screening for Canine Hip Dysplasia

Canine Hip Dysplasia (CHD) is the most common, heritable orthopedic problem seen in dogs. It affects virtually all breeds of dogs but is especially problematic in large and giant breeds. Clinically, the disease manifests itself in one of two ways: 1) a severe form that typically afflicts the younger animal and is usually characterized by marked pain and lameness or 2) a more chronic form with more gradual onset of clinical signs such as mild, intermittent pain, stiffness and restricted range of motion in the hips as the dog ages. In many cases, the chronic form may be clinically silent.

Breeders and veterinarians have long sought a reliable method to determine the likelihood of a dog developing CHD and passing that genetic trait to any offspring. It was generally recognized that the current diagnostic methods of hip evaluation were associated with disappointing progress in reducing the frequency of CHD. In 1983, Dr. Gail Smith, a veterinary orthopedic surgeon and bioengineer from the University of Pennsylvania School of Veterinarian Medicine, began to actively research and develop new scientific method for the early diagnosis of Canine Hip Dysplasia. Research in his laboratory resulted in a diagnostic method capable of estimating the susceptibility for CHD in populations of dogs as young as sixteen weeks. The method has shown distinct advantages over the standard CHD diagnostic method that evaluates dogs at two years or older. The University of Pennsylvania Hip Improvement Program (PennHIP) was founded as an extension of Dr. Smith's laboratory research. Below are answers to some commonly asked questions about PennHIP method.

What Exactly Is PennHIP?

PennHIP is a scientific method to evaluate a dog for its susceptibility to develop Hip Dysplasia. The radiographic procedure involves a special positioning of the dog so that the dog's "passive hip laxity" can be accurately measured. In simple terms, passive hip laxity refers to the degree of looseness of the hip ball in the hip socket when the dog's muscles are completely relaxed. Research has shown that the degree of passive hip laxity is an important factor in determining susceptibility to develop Degenerative Joint Disease (DJD) later in life. Radiographic evidence of hip DJD also known as osteoarthritis, is the universally accepted confirmation of CHD. PennHIP is being marketed by International Canine Genetics, Inc. (ICG) of Malvern, PA.

How Was PennHIP Developed?

The development of PennHIP has involved multiple disciplines including biomechanics, orthopedics, clinical medicine, radiology, epidemiology and population genetics. The first phase of development involved sophisticated biomechanical testing to determine the optimal patient position for measuring hip laxity. By monitoring passive hip laxity in dogs as they matured, it was discovered that hip laxity was the primary factor in the development of the DJD characteristic of CHD. That is, the radiographic expression of DJD was statistically significantly correlated with the degree of measured passive hip laxity. In addition, the CHD prediction was shown to be acceptably accurate in populations of puppies as young as sixteen weeks of age. Moreover, the correlation between passive hip laxity and subsequent hip DJD was shown to increase over the four-month figures when hips were evaluated at six months and twelve months of age. In the same studies, it was shown that there was no statistically significant correlation between laxity and DJD when the standard hip extended view was used. In addition, no other method used to evaluate for CHD has undergone similar rigorous testing through controlled scientific studies to determine diagnostic accuracy.

How Does PennHIP Differ from Evaluation Methods Which Use the Hip Extended Position?

PennHIP differs in some very fundamental and important ways. First, PennHIP was developed and tested following strict scientific protocol and the results of these studies have been published (and continue to be) in peer-reviewed, scientific journals. More than a decade of research and analysis has produced a body of information in support of PennHIP's effectiveness. As with all diagnostic tests, PennHIP's accuracy is not 100 percent, but in direct comparisons it is far superior to any other available diagnostic method. Second, passive hip laxity is objectively measured and the resulting Hip Evaluation Report is not issued in a pass/fail framework. PennHIP specifically measures passive joint laxity and includes the quantitative measurement in its report. Based on the degree of laxity, the individual dog is then ranked relative to other members of the same breed. (Note: Breed specific rankings are given when there are twenty or more evaluations. If there are fewer than twenty evaluations — ranking is made to the general dog population.) For example, a dog receiving a ranking in the 70th percentile means that thirty percent of its breed members have hips that are tighter. This allows breeders to easily identify the animals with tighter hips within each breed. As shown in our studies, dogs with tighter hips are less likely to develop CHD and pass that genetic tendency on to future generations. Third, because PennHIP is measuring maximal passive hip laxity, the position of the patients is very different from the hip-extended position. The hip-extended position has been used for more than thirty years to screen hips for either DJD, laxity or both. Laboratory studies, however, have indicated wide diagnostic variability among radiologists in interpreting this view. Further, through biomechanical testing, the hip-extended view was found to mask the underlying true joint laxity and through direct comparison, the predictive value for CHD was shown to be inferior to the PennHIP procedure. Most importantly, the heritability of the diseased phenotype scored in the hip-extended view has not been studied in most breeds of dogs. A knowledge of heritability is critical to determine whether selection pressure will produce genetic change. Estimates for the heritability of passive hip laxity drawn from analysis of full pedigrees for the breeds examined thus far in the studies show high values (for German Shepherd Dogs, heritability = 0.61). Fourth, the PennHIP method is based on strict quality control. To take PennHIP radiographs, veterinarians must undergo training and a certification process to demonstrate competency. The data generated from PennHIP undergoes regular review and statistical analysis so that useful information, by breed, is available to judge progress toward reducing CHD. For optimal validity, it is mandatory that all PennHIP radiographs be submitted for analysis and inclusion in the PennHIP database. This policy eliminates the practice of prescreening radiographs and sending only the best for evaluation, resulting in biased hip data for any given breed.

What Happens to My Dog During a PennHIP Evaluation?

To obtain diagnostic radiographs, it is important that the patient and the surrounding hip musculature be completely relaxed. For the comfort and safety of the animal, this requires sedation, however, some veterinarians prefer general anesthesia. Typically, three separate radiographs are made during an evaluation. The first is a compression view where the femurs are positioned in a neutral, stance-phase orientation and the femoral heads are pushed fully into the sockets. This helps show the true depth of the hip socket and gives an indication of the "fit" of the ball in the socket. The second radiograph is the distraction view. Again, the hips are positioned in a neutral orientation and a special positioning device is used to apply a harmless force to cause the hips to displace laterally. This position is the most accurate and sensitive for showing the degree of passive laxity. Passive laxity has been shown to correlate with the susceptibility to develop DJD. A hip extended view is also included for the sole purpose of examining for any existing joint disease such as osteoarthritis. The PennHIP procedure has been safely performed on thousands of patients.

What Is the Cost of Having My Dog Evaluated?

The total fee for a PennHIP evaluation is determined by the veterinarian providing the service. It is important to remember that the total service includes sedation/anesthesia, three radiographs, office consultation and all charges associated with mailing and film evaluation. You will not find it necessary to write a separate check for evaluation fees or mailing your dog's films. The veterinarian performing the procedure is responsible for payment and film submission. The film evaluation charge will be included in the total cost of a PennHIP evaluation.

Is PennHIP Going To Replace Other Commercially Available Systems?

As technology advances, the veterinary professional community will offer and utilize improved methods of disease diagnosis. The dog breeding community will also endorse those methods that help them achieve their goals of reducing the frequency of hip dysplasia in dogs while maintaining other desirable traits and features. The PennHIP technology and research have been and will continue to be, fully presented to the veterinary medical community for its review. PennHIP has been received enthusiastically as a major step toward reducing the frequency of CHD. We encourage and welcome continued scientific examination and comparison of PennHIP to any available or new methods of canine hip dysplasia diagnosis.

Will AKC and Other Breed Registration Organizations "Recognize" PennHIP?

ICG is working with many organizations to present the PennHIP technology and the positive impact it holds for reducing Canine Hip Dysplasia. It is conceivable that at some point a PennHIP reference might be included as part of the dog's registry information. However, all hip evaluation reports are considered confidential medical information and are released only to the PennHIP veterinarian and the owner of the dog (unless the owner requests otherwise).

How Does This Benefit Me as an Owner or Breeder of Dogs?

Scientific data confirms that the PennHIP method surpasses other diagnostic methods in the ability to accurately predict susceptibility to developing CHD. The method can be performed on dogs as young as sixteen weeks of age compared with two years using the standard technique. The ability to receive an early estimate of a dog's hip integrity is important whether the dog's intended purpose will be for breeding, for working or as a family pet. The data generated by PennHIP will allow breeders to confidently identify the members of their breeding stock with the tightest hips. The PennHIP interpretation will also permit breeders to assess the progress they are making with their breeding program as they strive to reduce the amount of hip laxity in their dogs. Pet owners are able to assess their pet's risk of developing CHD and make lifestyle adjustments for their dog, if necessary, to enhance the quality of their pet's life.

How Can I Get the Name of a PennHIP Veterinarian or Get Answers to Additional Questions?

To obtain the name of a veterinarian near you who is trained and certified to perform the PennHIP procedure, call ICG at (800) 248-8099. If there is not a veterinarian near you presently, additional veterinarians are being trained throughout the country. If your veterinarian would like to learn more about PennHIP, please have him/her contact ICG directly.

International Canine Genetics, Inc.
271 Great Valley Parkway
Malvern, PA 19355
Phone: (610) 640-1244 or (800) 248-8099
Fax: (610) 640-5754.

Chapter 14

Infectious Diseases

by Denise Juppé

With proper care and feeding, most pets lead lives that are healthy and problem free. But as with humans, almost every pet will fall sick occasionally, despite the best care. Some pet diseases can be transmitted to humans, though preventative measures can be taken which will help minimize the risk of being infected by a sick animal.

This chapter will discuss some of the diseases which may affect pets, and which could be passed on to humans as well. It will consider the special case of people who are "immuno-compromised," whose immune systems are weakened, whether because of old age, AIDS, cancer, diabetes or other factors. Finally it will outline preventative measures, both for pets which may be permanent members of your facility and for your pet visitors.

Nature doesn't often fit into our neat categories, so even though the diseases covered here are grouped by species, there will be some overlap. Some diseases are strongly associated with a certain group of animals, but can be infectious for others. Where this is important, it will be noted.

Diseases Common to Dogs and Cats

Rabies

Of all the diseases that can be transmitted from animals to people, rabies is probably best known. Though long associated with dogs, there are actually more cases diagnosed in cats. In the present day, outdoor cats do a lot more hunting than dogs. This provides them a greater exposure to wildlife diseases. Wildlife accounts for 90% of rabies cases seen it the US. Why then do we vaccinate our dogs and cats against rabies? Because once they do get rabies, they're statistically likely to expose five times as many people to the virus as a wild animal would. Rabies is a viral disease, which means that it cannot be cured using antibiotics. Vaccination (usually every two years) is a vital part of pet care for dogs and cats.

Salmonella

Though people usually think of salmonella as a type of food poisoning, it is also a common infectious disease of animals, especially young ones. Turtles, once kept as pets by many children, were banned in the US when it became apparent that they were a significant source of Salmonella related illness. Salmonella is still the second most common cause of bacterial diarrhea in the US and, though most people do get it from eating contaminated food, those at risk (infants, older adults, the immunocompromised) should be careful when handling pets. Hand washing is one very simple way of lowering the chances of infection. Puppies and kittens with diarrhea should, of course, be seen by a veterinarian for evaluation and kept away from those at high risk for infection until they are well again. Pets should be fed good quality pet food and/or completely cooked foods, as they run the same risk of infection from undercooked foods as humans. For a more detailed discussion of prevention, see the section on *Prevention for the Immunocompromised.*

Campylobacter

Like Salmonella, Campylobacter is frequently assumed to be an infection caused by food poisoning and, indeed, in most cases contaminated food is the culprit. However, dogs and cats, especially young animals and those who have been living in crowded animal shelter conditions, are at risk for catching and transmitting the Campylobacter bacteria. In humans, Campylobacter causes acute diarrhea, sometimes with blood or mucus mixed in. It is successfully treated with antibiotics. Hand washing, as well as prompt treatment and isolation of a sick pet, are the best lines of defense against spreading this disease.

Dog and Cat Bites

Every year, about one million people are bitten by dogs or cats in the US. While most of these bites are trivial, bite wounds account for about 1% of all emergency room visits! One half to two-thirds of those bitten are children, probably because on the whole they have more contact than adults with pets.

The mouths of healthy cats and dogs contain a wide spectrum of bacteria. Only a few kinds are responsible for most infections contracted by people. If someone at your facility is bitten, it is important that the wound be *thoroughly* cleaned and disinfected. Dog bites are more common, but cat bites are more likely to become infected because cats tend to inflict deeper, more puncture-type wounds. A person who has been bitten should consult a doctor about beginning a course of antibiotics if s/he falls into one or more of the following categories: older than 50, bitten on the hands or face, bitten by a cat, diabetic or immunocompromised. If no antibiotics are administered, the wound should be watched for signs of infection (redness, soreness, swelling, pus) for 24-48 hours after the bite. The rabies vaccination history of the animal should be obtained. A tetanus shot should be administered to the bitten person if it's been more than 10 years since his/her last one.

Dogs

There are few diseases that are unique to dogs and transmissible to humans, but there are two parasites of dogs, ticks and worms, that are potentially troublesome for our species as well as canines. The watchword for both these problems is "vigilance." Taking proper precautions will go a long way towards eliminating these undesirable "guests."

Tick-borne diseases

Ticks are parasites of warm-blooded animals, capable of transmitting several diseases to their hosts as they feed. These diseases aren't passed on directly from dog to man, for instance, but ticks are mobile little creatures. They can "jump" from one host to another, thus they are capable of infecting a person who has been handling a dog. Because dogs and people are likely to walk through tick habitats (primarily woods and grasslands), it is a very good idea to check both after such excursions, particularly in the summer months. There are several types of ticks, so you should try to acquaint yourself with which kinds are most common in your area. The most common diseases caused by ticks are

a) **Rocky Mountain Spotted Fever** — oddly enough, a problem found more often in the Southeastern US than in the Rocky Mountains. The symptoms are not well defined. There is fever, often (but not always) a rash on the palms of the hands and soles of the feet, muscle soreness and headaches. Can be serious if not treated early.

b) **Lyme Disease** — a disease first described just 20 years ago, it has become the most frequently reported tick disease in the US. It is usually caused by the deer tick, which is very small and difficult to detect. Often there is a target-type rash around the bite. Fever, stiffness and rash may be present in the patient. Arthritis-like symptoms appear in later stages.

c) **Erlichiosis** — can be confused with Rocky Mountain Spotted Fever and Lyme Disease. The symptoms are very unspecific, i.e., fever, headache and malaise. Rare, but can be serious or fatal.

All of these are bacterial infections which are treated with antibiotics, the earlier the better. There is another condition, "Tick Paralysis," which is caused by a toxin secreted by the tick. Once the tick is removed, paralysis of the patient gradually disappears.

Worms

Worms are a *much* greater health hazard for dogs than they are for humans. Two of the worms mentioned below (tapeworms and heart worms) can infect people, but only live in their human hosts as cysts, doing little harm. Only the roundworm can produce any significant symptoms in people, with children being the most likely to contract them. Roundworm eggs, which are excreted and then contaminate soil, must be ingested in order to cause disease. Children, through outdoor play, are more likely to come in contact with sources of infection.

Heart worm: A serious but preventable infection for dogs, who should be routinely wormed to avoid problems.

Tapeworm: Once considered quite rare in the US, the latest findings are that it is spreading among foxes and coyotes in the northern Plains states and Texas. This could become more of a problem for dogs in coming years. It is spread to humans through contact with infected soil, hands, clothing, food and flies.

Roundworms: Pups and kittens are subject to a very high rate of infection from roundworms. Bitches can pass the worms on to the pups in the womb or while nursing. Queens (female cats) can only pass them on while nursing. Very young animals are generally confined to a rather small space which can become heavily infested with roundworm eggs. Also, most new animals aren't seen by a vet until they're 6 to 8 weeks old.

For these reasons, people handling very young animals are at risk of becoming infected with roundworms unless they wash their hands thoroughly afterwards. If you acquire a very young animal, be sure that it is seen by a vet. Roundworms, known more formally as *toxocaral larva migrans*, or TLM, is still not a common human disease, affecting maybe 1000 people a year. Three-quarters of these infections are in the eyes. A more severe type of roundworm infection, originating in raccoons, is discussed below.

Cats

Toxoplasmosis

Pregnant women have long been warned about the risk of contracting toxoplasmosis from household cats, which could lead to serious neurological damage for babies born with the infection. While the risk is real, the true picture is a little more complicated. Toxoplasmosis is widespread among humans and other warm-blooded animals. In fact, 30-40% of all adults have antibodies to it in their bloodstream. This means that they've been exposed to it sometime earlier in their lives. Uncooked meat is often a source of the infection; it's where most cats acquire it in the first place.

Toxoplasmosis is caused by a protozoon, a one-celled animal, so it can't be cured with antibiotics. Many people will only have mild, flu-like symptoms or none at all. The exception is among AIDS patients and the immunocompromised, for whom any infection can be devastating. It is thought that these people are usually experiencing the reactivation of a latent infection, rather than a new infection acquired from a cat in their present environment. Nevertheless, both pregnant women and people with lowered immunity should avoid changing cat litter, wear gloves when gardening, wash their hands after handling raw meat and wash vegetables. Cats should never be fed raw meat or be allowed to scavenge in garbage cans. Work is being done towards the development of a vaccine, but none are yet ready for commercial use.

Cat scratch disease

So called "cat scratch disease" is caused by a bacteria in the family *Bartonella*. Because it has been determined that there are other routes besides cat scratches that can cause the disease, it is now officially designated "Bartonellosis." It is *generally* transmitted by cat (and especially kitten) scratches or, possibly, the bite of infected fleas. Most people who are scratched don't develop infections; most infections that do develop are not serious and require no treatment. A small fraction of cases do become serious, as the bacteria infect the blood stream. These are treated with antibiotics. People who are immunocompromised are, not surprisingly, at a greater risk for developing these infections. Much about the origins and treatment of Bartonellosis is not yet well understood or is controversial. Cat scratches should be cleaned and observed for signs of infection.

Feline sporotrichosis

Cats that develop open sores (ulcers) should be taken to a veterinarian. Extreme care should be taken to avoid coming in contact with the sores. Sporotrichosis is a fungus, it is uncommon in humans, but is also easily transmitted from cats to people. This fungus presents a greater hazard for the immunocompromised, who may develop a systemic form of the disease after exposure.

A note on cats and rodent disease

The Hanta virus and bubonic plague are two very serious diseases that are found in rodents. They are quite rare in the human population. Because cats are hunters, there is a small chance of their playing a part in bringing humans into contact with these diseases. In the case of the Hanta virus, steps should be taken to keep cats from bringing rodents indoors. All wild rodents, dead or alive, should be removed from human dwellings with extreme care.

Bubonic plague, reported mostly in the western states of the US, is carried by both rodents and their fleas. Cats can become infected with plague through contact with either. Plague differs from Hanta because it is a bacterial infection and can be treated with antibiotics. It is still a serious disease. It can be spread quickly into human populations, particularly in the form of plague pneumonia. It is best to know if there is plague in your area, but any cat that develops swelling on its body and seems listless and feverish should be taken to a vet promptly.

Raccoons

Baylisascaris

Taking a cute little baby raccoon out of the woods and making it a pet is a *not* a good idea. This is probably not an option that you've considered for your pet therapy program, anyway. Knowing that raccoons can harbor a type of roundworm that is infectious for many warm-blooded animals, including humans, may make them seem less appealing. It is estimated that up to 70-90% of young raccoons in the northern part of the US are infected (the prevalence is much lower in the South). Once considered a relatively rare disease, it is now thought that this roundworm is the most common cause of *larval migrans* (see Dogs, above) in warm-blooded animals and a significant health threat to humans. Roundworm eggs must be ingested to cause disease, but they can survive for months on infected food, soil, clothing, cages and any other materials contaminated with feces of pets or wild raccoons.

The most relevant information for pet owners is the finding that young dogs can become infected with these roundworms, thus increasing the potential for transmission to humans. Worming medicine used to prevent dog roundworms is equally effective for *Baylisascaris*. It is important that dogs be routinely wormed and that their stools be examined once a year.

Rabbits

Tularemia

If a pet rabbit becomes listless, with loss of appetite and possible fever, it should be checked out by the vet for a possible Tularemia infection. Tularemia is a bacterial infection of warm-blooded animals, to which rabbits and humans are especially susceptible. Ticks are important in its transmission. Humans may contract it after contact with infected rabbits (during hunting season, for example), via ticks and, occasionally, a dog or cat bite. Dogs and cats are occasionally infected with it, through eating dead rabbits, through ticks or fly bites or through drinking contaminated water. The infection is bacterial. It can be a serious disease in humans if left untreated.

Birds

Chlamydiosis
Any bird which seems overtly ill, with symptoms such as diarrhea, poor appetite, low energy (depression) and ruffled feathers, should be evaluated by a vet for this infection. Birds who have been stressed by crowded conditions during shipment or changes in environment or diet, are especially susceptible. Chlamydia is a bacterial infection which can be transmitted to people through the air, that is, by breathing it in. People will respond quite differently, some developing what appears to be a chronic cold, while others may develop an infection severe enough to warrant hospitalization. Antibiotics will clear the infection in humans and birds.

Prevention

What can you do to prevent your pet therapy animal, your patients and yourself from contracting any of these diseases? As was noted at the beginning of this chapter, there are a number of very simple precautions that you can take which will go a long way towards keeping humans and their pets disease-free.

If you are keeping a pet at or for your facility on a permanent basis, you should provide it with routine veterinary care. This means:

a) a yearly checkup (more for younger animals)
b) a vaccination program appropriate for your type of pet

c) worming, in the case of a dog, on a schedule determined by your vet

Whoever is responsible for the care of the animal should also ensure that s/he is doing the following:
a) feeding the pet good quality pet food and clean water
b) regularly inspecting for ticks, if the pet is a dog, as well as inspecting dogs and humans after visits to woods or meadow lands
c) taking care that cats don't eat small wild animals or scavenge garbage cans
d) taking any sick animal to the vet for prompt treatment and isolating the animal until it is well again

Do NOT make pets of wild animals. If you have an outdoor cat as a pet, do not take on the removal of any small dead animal if the cat ever brings one indoors. Call your local Animal Control for assistance.

Anyone handling pets should be encouraged to **wash their hands thoroughly** before and afterwards, as a matter of good hygiene and as very effective tool for preventing the spread of disease.

If you do not have a resident pet, but rely on visits from the outside, then a simple set of guidelines for pet visits should be implemented. All potential pet visitors should be

a) free of obvious symptoms of disease
b) up to date on vaccines and worming (if appropriate)
c) from a reputable facility or organization, one with clean and uncrowded facilities and which cares well for its inhabitants

If you are involved at a facility where some patients are immunocompromised, please read the next section.

Prevention for the Immunocompromised

Mention has been made throughout this chapter of diseases which are of greater concern to those whose immune systems have been weakened by disease, age or certain medical treatments. It should be pointed out that there are several levels of immune system dysfunction. The aged are often mildly immuno-compromised, but people with diabetes, some cancers, liver cirrhosis, who are HIV-positive or have had marrow or organ transplants, all have immune systems which may be functioning far below normal. Finally, people diagnosed with "full blown" AIDS (whose T-cell count has fallen below 200) have great difficulties in fighting off opportunistic infections, as their bodies can no longer manufacture the cells which will help to fight them off.

For most people who are considered immunocompromised, taking the precautions outlined under the *Prevention* section above will be sufficient for avoiding serious disease. Even in this population, the prevalence of diseases caught from companion animals is thought to be quite low. Pets should be given all recommended vaccinations, taken to the vet for a yearly exam and at the earliest sign of illness and fed only a diet of high quality commercial pet food. Patients should wash their hands thoroughly before and after handling pets, wear gloves when gardening and avoid cleaning litter boxes, bird cages or aquariums.

When choosing a pet, those who are immunocompromised or who work with them, may wish to avoid picking a very young one. Young animals, especially those with diarrhea, are much more likely to be disease carriers. Once chosen, the animal should have a complete veterinary exam to assure that it's in good health when being introduced into the household or facility.

Many of the diseases that may be passed on by pets can also be acquired from other sources, with the possible exception of Bartonella (cat scratch disease). Tuberculosis *could* be contracted from a pet, but is much more likely to come from exposure to another person. Cryptosporidium, Giardia, Salmonella and

Campylobacter are diseases which are more often acquired from food and water supplies. The immunocompromised person should be sure to wash up after handling uncooked meat and cook meat and eggs thoroughly before consuming them. Though they can be contracted from other sources, the most *likely* diseases to be contracted from pets are Salmonella and Campylobacter, simply because they are so common.

Dogs are usually less fastidious about grooming themselves than cats and therefore slightly more likely to transmit Campylobacter or Salmonella infections. For severely immunocompromised patients, kennels and dog shows are a risk, as kennel cough (Bordetella) can be transmitted to humans. Others should be sure to have their dog vaccinated for Bordetella before placing him/her in a kennel.

People who are immunocompromised are often warned against keeping birds, but most infections in birds are not contagious to humans. Contact with wild birds, including pigeons, should be avoided as they are more likely than domestic birds to be harboring Campylobacter or Salmonella.

Reptiles should NOT be kept by immunocompromised patients, they have very high rates for carrying Salmonella. Hamsters and gerbils are as likely as dogs and cats to carry Salmonella, Camylobacter and Giardia; they should be handled and their cages cleaned with the same care as other mammals.

Finally, there are several brochures available to those seeking to minimize the risks of infections from pets to the immunocompromised. One California-based organization, PAWS (Pets Are Wonderful Support), publishes a variety, which include *Safe Pet Guidelines, Toxoplasmosis and Your Cat, Zoonoses and Your Bird* and *Cat Scratch Disease.* (See *Organizations* in the *Appendix.*) With proper care and handling, a pet can provide great psychological and emotional support for all patients, with very little risk of causing disease.

Chapter 15

Death of a Pet

How Will I Deal With My Residents' Grief When A Facility Pet Dies?

More and more, the topic of grief over the loss of a pet is being written and talked about, as we become more aware of the fact that it is a very real emotion which must be dealt with. This loss is a major one in a pet owner's life. When we lose a facility pet, the residents lose the unconditional love that they have shared together. They will miss the animal, its kisses and cuddles, its humorous antics and, most of all, its presence.

Now that Prancer has been in the Masonic Home for over four years, residents look forward to seeing him. Everyone knows he follows me everywhere. If he is not with me, visitors, residents, volunteers and staff alike ask questions like, "Where's your shadow?" or "Why isn't Prancer here today?" or "I hope Prancer isn't sick today?"

As with any loss that occurs, your residents will go through several stages during the grieving process. These stages are, in order, shock, anger, sadness, guilt and, finally, acceptance.

Gloria J. Roettger MS, a counselor in private practice in Olympia, Washington, specializes in pet loss. She writes, "Another stage I find specific to the loss of a pet is the memory phase. This lasts long after the pet has died and involves remembering very special times together with that pet and the uniqueness of its personality. People often have many special stories to tell of the pet and its significance to their lives."

In my facility, with the untimely death of our six-month-old Golden Retriever, Moses, people who loved him experienced all the stages of grief. Men and women alike shed tears of sadness over his loss. They asked over and over how it had happened and why it had happened. They were saddened by his absence. Men in our wood shop who had grown very attached to him needed hugs and time to shed tears as they recalled how much they had grown to love him. His passing was handled in much the same way as the passing of our residents; a memo was posted on the bulletin boards and an "In Memorial" was placed in our newspaper, **Home Team**. Moses' picture was published in the **Home Team** along with the following poem:

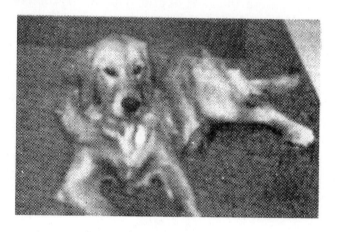

A Bargain Pup
By Garnett Ann Schultz

I bought a pup with wagging tail,
Two trusting eyes that never fail,
A bit of fluff — an outstretched paw,
Real loyalty — without a flaw;
And though the price was small would seem,
He came equipped with shining dreams.
I bought a pup, a tiny life,
Some love within a world of strife.
Devotion such as none I'd known,
He changed my house into a home;

Forever waiting for me there,
Affection that he longs to share.
He changes not though I may frown,
I know he'll never let me down.
He listens when I care to speak,
'Tis only love that he would seek.
He doesn't care for wealth or fame,
Delights to hear me call his name.
The price I paid was small indeed
For happiness to fill a need,
For understanding, warmth so true,
The greatest friend I ever knew,
A wagging tail, a trust complete,
My puppy — waiting at my feet.

My husband and I personally received sympathy cards from residents and friends alike. We were also supported by our church family who knew of our work with therapy dogs.

Moses passed away the weekend before Thanksgiving. We were very fortunate because Jackie and Jerry Pentel of Golden Haven Golden Retrievers in Denton, Maryland, the breeders from whom we had purchased Moses, had another litter that would be ready for their new homes on December 20, 1992, a Sunday. Because of our tragic and untimely loss, they were kind enough to make our request for a puppy a top priority. They chose a pup with the best temperament for our needs. Nicholas arrived home on Sunday night and after a trip to the vet on Monday morning he began his new life as a facility pet.

Nicky's arrival was also announced through memos on the facility's bulletin boards and with an article and a prayer in our **Home Team** newspaper. The article and prayer read:

"As most of you know by now, our newest addition to the department is *Nicholas*, affectionately known as 'Nicky.' Nicky joins his brothers King, Bandit and Prancer at the Abdill household and has won the hearts of our residents as our latest therapy dog.

He's lovable, fluffy and has already learned to sit and come on command."

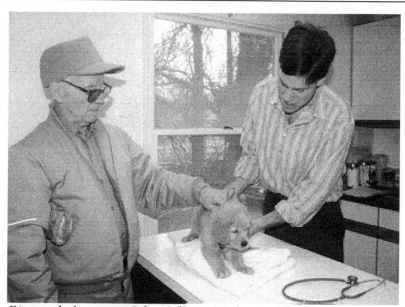

Pictured above are John Gilbert, Nicky and Dr. Larry Wolf, VMD, as Nicky receives his official check-up and Health Certificate on Monday, December 21, 1992, at the Willingboro Veterinary Clinic

As we have worked with Pet Therapy and gained a better perspective of its benefits to our Masonic Home residents, we must not forget the welfare of the pets involved in such a program. This prayer might well represent the thoughts of all dogs whether therapy dogs or family pets.

If the loss of a pet in your program occurs, the issue of grief must be addressed. It is important to remember that your pet touched your residents' lives in many ways — some that you will never know about. The loss needs to be acknowledged and the stages of grief shared. Be willing to talk about the pet and share in the "memory stage" of grief. Be willing to talk about the pet and how wonderful he or she was. Keep in mind that you are the facilitator of this program from its introduction to its closure.

Additional information on grief can be obtained from the following sources:

Carmock, Betty J., EdD. RN. 1991. "Pet Loss and the Elderly." *Holistic Nursing Practice.* 1991:5(2):80-87: Aspen Publishing, Inc.

Delta Society, 289 Perimeter Road East, Renton, WA 98055-1329, (800) 869-6898

Kelly, Diane, PhD. 1989. "Coping With Grief." *Cat Fancy* (February, 1989), pp. 55.

Rosenberg, Marc A., VMD. 1986. "Death of the Family Pet...Losing a Family Friend." Adapted by the ALPO Veterinary Advisory Panel from the monograph, *Companion Animal Loss and Pet Owner Grief.* ALPO Pet Center. Write: ALPO Professional Relations, PO Box 25200, Lehigh Valley, PA 18002-5200

Swift, W. Brad, DVM. 1987. "Coping with Pet Loss." *Cat Fancy* (March, 1987), pp. 17.

A DOG'S PRAYER
By Beth Norman Harris

Treat me kindly, my beloved master, for no heart in all the world is more grateful for kindness than this loving heart of mine.

Do not break my spirit with a stick, for though I would lick your hand between the blows, your patience and understanding will more quickly teach me the things you would have me do.

Speak to me often, for your voice is the world's sweetest music, as you must know by the fierce wagging of my tail when your footstep falls upon my waiting ear.

When it is cold and wet, please take me inside for now I am a domesticated animal, no longer used to bitter elements. And I ask no greater glory than the privilege of sitting at your feet beside the hearth.

Though had you no home, I would rather follow you through ice and snow than rest upon the softest pillow in the warmest home in all the land, for you are my God and I am the devoted worshipper.

Keep my pan filled with fresh water, for although I should not reproach you were it dry, I cannot tell you when I suffer thirst.

Feed me clean food that I may stay well, to romp and play and do your bidding, to walk by your side and stand ready, willing and able protect you with my life should your life be in danger.

And, beloved master, should the Great Master see fit to deprive me of my health or sight, do not turn me away from you. Rather hold me gently in your arms as skilled hands grant me the merciful boon of eternal rest...and I will leave you knowing with the last breath I draw, my fate was ever safest in your hands.

Amen.

If the Burden is Too Heavy

Veterinary teaching institutions, in studying the human-companion animal bond, are increasing their efforts to help pet owners cope with lingering grief. Some of the teaching institutions have social workers who are specially trained to counsel pet owners. Among the most well known programs are those at:

The Animal Medical Center
New York City   (212) 838-8100

The University of Pennsylvania
School of Veterinary Medicine
Philadelphia, Pennsylvania   (215) 898-4525

University of California
School of Veterinary Medicine
Davis, California (916) 752-7418

University of Minnesota
College of Veterinary Medicine
St. Paul, Minnesota   (612) 624-4747

Colorado State University
College of Veterinary Medicine
Fort Collins, Colorado   (303) 221-4535

Washington State University
College of Veterinary Medicine
Pullman, Washington   (509) 335-1297

University of Florida
College of Veterinary Medicine
Gainesville, Florida
Pet Support Hotline (904) 392-4700, ext. 4080

Finally, should grief become an unexpected part of your pet therapy program, perhaps these words can help you and your residents through the pain:

"Like all vets I hated doing this, painless though it was, but to me there has always been a comfort in the knowledge that the last thing these helpless animals knew was the sound of a friendly voice and the touch of a gentle hand."
— James Herriot
All Things Wise and Wonderful
Copyright 1977, St. Martin's Press, New York

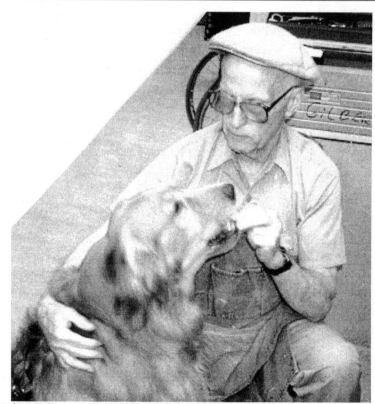

John Gilbert takes a break from his work in the woodshop to spend a moment with Nicky

Chapter 16

Policies and Procedures

Developing Individual Policies

Once it has been decided that a program is feasible and the "go ahead" has been given, the next step is to develop policies and procedures. A word of caution here: be realistic and do not try to do it all (something Activity Professionals are famous for!). Also consider possible turf wars that might occur. What other departments, such as housekeeping, nursing and/or social services, need to be involved and what might they see as their role in the program? Don't write policies and procedures that concern them without consulting them first. Determine what they are actually willing to do in the implementation of this program.

Try to develop policies and procedures that are practical, helpful and realistic. Their purpose is to outline precisely what needs to be done, when, how, where and by whom. They should be written so that anyone can understand them and so as to ensure that the program can be carried out even in your absence. Although it is certainly not possible to think of everything at the beginning, do your best and remember that policies or procedures can always be amended or updated if you find there are more considerations to be taken into account.

Sample regulations from New Jersey and policies and procedures for the Masonic Home of New Jersey are shown in this chapter.

New Jersey Standards For Licensure Of Long-Term Care Facilities

Guidelines And Considerations For Pet Facilitated Therapy In New Jersey Institutions are shown below. Because regulations for each state are different, those of New Jersey are included only as a guideline. Contact your own state's Department of Health for their current regulations.

I. **All Pets**
    A. Companion pets should not pose a threat or nuisance to the patients, staff or visitors because of size, odor, sound, disposition or behavioral characteristics. Aggressive or unprovoked threatening behavior should mandate the pet's immediate removal.
    B. Animals which may be approved include: dogs, cats, birds (except carnivorous), fish, hamsters, gerbils, guinea pigs and domestic rabbits. Wild animals such as turtles and other reptiles, ferrets and carnivorous birds should not be permitted in the program.
    C. In order to participate, dogs or cats should be either altered or determined not to be in estrus ("heat").
    D. Sanitary constraints:
        1. Pets will be prohibited from the following areas:
            a) food preparation, storage and serving areas, with the exception of participating resident's bedroom;
            b) areas used for the cleaning or storage of human food utensils and dishes;
            c) vehicles used for the transportation of prepared food;
            d) nursing stations, drug preparation areas, sterile and clean supply rooms;
            e) linen storage areas;
            f) areas where soiled or contaminated materials are stored.

2. Food handlers should not be involved in the cleanup of animal waste.

3. The administrator is responsible for acceptable pet husbandry practices and may delegate specific duties to any other staff members except food handlers. The areas of responsibility include: feeding and watering, food cleanup/cage cleaning, exercising and grooming.

4. Spilling or scattering of food and water should not lessen the standard of housekeeping or contribute to an increase in vermin or objectionable odor.

5. Dogs and cats must be effectively housebroken and provisions made for suitably disposing of their body wastes.

6. Animal waste should be disposed of in a manner which prevents the material from becoming a community health or nuisance problem and in accordance with applicable sanitation rules and ordinances. Accepted methods include disposal in sealed plastic bags (utilizing municipally approved trash removal systems) or via the sewage system for feces.

7. Proper and frequent hand washing shall be a consideration of all persons handling animals.

E. Animals found to be infested with external parasites (ticks, fleas or lice) or which shows signs of illness (for example, vomiting or diarrhea) should be immediately removed from the premises and taken to the facility's veterinarian.

F. The parent or guardian of a child bitten by a dog, cat or other animal, when no physician attends such a child, shall, within 12 hours after first having knowledge that the child was so bitten, report to the person designated by law or by local board, under authority of law, to receive reports of reportable communicable diseases in the municipality in which the child so bitten may be the name, age, sex, color and precise location of the child (N.J.R.S. 26:4-80). If an adult is bitten by a dog, cat or other animal and no physician attends him, the adult, or, if he is incapacitated, the person caring for him, shall report to the person designated by law or local board of health to receive reports of communicable diseases in the municipality in which the adult so bitten may be the name, age, sex, color and the precise location of the adult. The report shall be made within 12 hours after the adult was so bitten (N.J.S.A. 26:4-81).

G. The local health department must be promptly notified by telephone of any pet which dies on the premises.

　1. If the deceased is a bird, the body should be immediately taken to the facility's veterinarian. If the veterinarian is not available, the deceased bird should be securely wrapped in impermeable wrapping material and frozen until veterinary consultation is available. Payment for a laboratory examination should be the responsibility of the institution or the pet's owner.

　2. If the deceased is another type of animal, the body should not be disposed until it is determined by the local department of health that rabies testing is not necessary.

H. The rights of residents who do not wish to participate in the pet program must be considered first. Patients not wishing to be exposed to animals should have available a pet free area within the participating facility.

II. Visiting Pets

A. Visiting pets are defined as any animal brought into the facility on a periodic basis for pet therapy purposes. The owner should accompany the animal and be responsible for its behavior and activities while it is visiting at the facility.

B. Visiting dogs should:

　1. be restricted to the areas designated by the facility administrator;

　2. maintain current vaccination against canine disease of distemper, hepatitis, leptospirosis, parainfluenza, parvovirus, coronavirus, bordetella (kennel cough) and

rabies. Proof of vaccination shall be included on a health certificate which is signed by a licensed veterinarian and kept on file at the facility;

3. be determined not to be in estrus ("heat") at the time of the visit;
4. be licensed and wear an identification tag on the collar, choke chain or harness, stating the dog's name, the owner's name, address and telephone number; and
5. be housebroken if more than four months of age. Younger dogs may be admitted subject to the approval of the administrator.

C. Visiting cats should:
1. Maintain current vaccination against feline pneumonitis, panleukopenia, rhinothraceitis, calcivirus, chlamydia and rabies. Proof of vaccination shall be included on a health certificate which is signed by a licensed veterinarian and kept on file at the facility.
2. Determined not to be in estrus ("heat") at the time of the visit.

D. Visiting hamsters, gerbils, guinea pigs, domestic rabbits, laboratory mice or rats:
1. The owner should be liable and responsible for the animal's activities and behavior.

E. No visiting birds should be allowed to participate in the program.

III. Residential Pets

A. Residential pets are defined as any animal which resides at a facility in excess of four hours during any calendar day and is owned by a staff member, patient, the facility or a facility approved party. The financial responsibility for the residential animal's maintenance is the animal owner's responsibility.
B. All documentation of compliance will be maintained by the facility administrator in a file for review and inspection.

The official health records should include the rabies
vaccination certificate and a current health certificate.

C. Residential animals should have a confinement area
separate from the patients where they can be restricted
when indicated. An area should be available for each
participating unit and should be approved by the
administrator.

D. A licensed veterinarian should be designated as the
facility's veterinarian and should be responsible for
establishing and maintaining a disease control program for
residential pets.

E. Specific Species:

1. Residential dogs should:

a) Maintain current vaccination against canine diseases
of distemper, hepatitis, letospirosis, parainfluenza,
parvovirus and rabies. In addition, the animal's file
should include a currently valid Rabies Vaccination
Certificate, NASPHV #51. A three year type rabies
vaccine should be utilized.

b) Have an annual heartworm test commencing at one
year of age and should be maintained on heartworm
preventative medication.

c) Have a fecal examination for internal parasites
twice yearly. Test results should be negative before
the dog's initial visit to the facility.

d) Follow the recommended procedures of the
facility's veterinarian for controlling external
parasites.

e) Be spayed/neutered.

f) Be licensed with the municipality and wear an
identification tag on the collar, choke chain or
harness, stating the dog's name, the owner's name,
address and telephone number.

g) Have a health certificate completed by a licensed
veterinarian within one week before the animal's

initial visit to the facility. The certificate should be updated annually thereafter.

h) Be immediately removed from the premises and taken to the facility's veterinarian if infested with internal or external parasites, vomit or have diarrhea or shows signs of a behavioral change or infectious disease. Medical records of the veterinarian's diagnosis and treatment should be maintained in the animal's file. The animal should not have patient contact until authorized by the facility's veterinarian.

i) Be housebroken if more than four months of age. Younger dogs may be admitted subject to the requirements of the administrator.

j) Be fed in accordance with the interval and quantity recommended by the facility's veterinarian. Feeding and watering bowls should be washed daily and stored separately from dishes and utensils used for human consumption.

k) Be provided fresh water daily and have 24-hour access to the water dish.

l) Be provided a suitable bedding area. Bedding should be cleaned or changed as needed. Dirty bedding should be processed or disposed of as necessary.

m) Be permitted outside the facility only if under the supervision of a staff member, a responsible person or within a fenced area.

n) Be regularly groomed and receive a bath whenever indicated.

2. Residential birds:

a) Should be treated by a licensed veterinarian with an approved chlortetracycline treatment regimen prior to being housed at the institution to ensure the absence of psittacosis. The period of treatment varies between 30 to 45 days and is species-dependent. A signed statement from the veterinarian indicating such treatment should be kept in the bird's file.

b) That die, or are suspected of having psittacosis, should be immediately taken to the facility's veterinarian. In the event the bird dies and the veterinarian is not available, the bird's body should be securely wrapped in impermeable wrapping material and frozen until veterinary consultation is available.

3. Residential hamsters, gerbils, guinea pigs, domestic rabbits, laboratory mice or rats:

a) Should be examined yearly by a licensed veterinarian for health status. A health certificate should be completed for each animal or group of animals. Any animal which becomes sick or dies should be promptly taken to the facility's veterinarian.

Masonic Home Of New Jersey Animal Assisted Therapy

Purpose: To enhance residents' quality of life through visual, physical, tactile, emotional and social stimulation.

Goals: Relative to animal assisted therapy:
1. increase self-esteem through the medium of unconditional love
2. stimulate play and movement
3. increase nurturing and provide joy
4. decrease or relieve depression by:
    a) watching – outdoor animals, fish tanks
    b) stroking – in-house visits
5. provide sensory stimulation
6. provide reality re-enforcement
7. encourage memory stimulation, reminiscing
8. provide therapeutic touch
9. increase social interaction:
    a) resident to resident
    b) resident to staff
    c) resident to volunteer
10. contribute to facility's "home-like" surroundings
11. provide experiences for, and stimulate life review
12. improve fine and gross motor skills
13. allow resident to make choices
14. provide expression of affection without consequence (patting, petting, hugging, kissing)

Selection: All residents may be included with the following exceptions:
- residents who express or show fear of animals
- residents with conflicting health diagnoses
- residents who do not wish to participate

Implementation: Animal assisted therapy techniques and activities

Pet Policies and Procedures:

1. General Requirements/Information
    a. The introduction of pets will not pose a threat or nuisance to the residents, staff or visitors because of size, color, odor, sound, disposition or behavioral characteristics. Aggressive or unprovoked threatening behavior will mandate the pet's immediate removal.
    b. Animals approved by the NJ Department of Institutions and which may be included by the Masonic Home of New Jersey include: dogs, cats, fish, Guinea pigs and rabbits. Any other species must first be approved by the Division of Licensing and Certification prior to acceptance by this facility. Approval by the administrator for any exception shall accompany all applications. If approved, subsequent current guidelines by the Division of Licensing and Certification must be followed.
    c. All dogs and cats must be determined not to be in estrus.
    d. All pets must be effectively controlled by leash, command, crate or tank.
    e. Either the parent/guardian of, or the person who has been bitten by a facility pet and not immediately attended by a physician, must report the incident within 12 hours. The report should include the name, age, sex, race and precise location of the person, and be made to the person designated by law, or by the local board under authority of law, to receive reports of communicable diseases in the municipality in which the person resides.
    f. If the facility becomes unable to provide adequate control or care of the pets, then the Pet Therapy program may, at the discretion of the administrator, his designees or a health officer, be revoked.

2. Sanitary Constraints
   a. Pets are prohibited from the following areas:
      1. food preparation, storage and serving areas
      2. areas used for cleaning or storage of utensils and dishes
      3. vehicles used for the transportation of prepared food
      4. employees' toilet, shower and dressing rooms
      5. nursing stations, drug preparation areas, sterile and clean supply rooms
      6. linen storage areas
      7. areas where soiled or contaminated materials are stored
   b. Food handlers shall not be involved in animal care and feeding or clean-up of animal food or waste.
   c. Spilling or scattering of food and water shall not lessen the standard of housekeeping or contribute to an increase of vermin or offensive odor.
3. Visiting Pets
   a. A visiting pet is defined as any animal brought into the facility for a period of less than four hours.
   b. No birds of any type are permitted in this Home.
   c. All pets must have current inoculations against the diseases particular to their species in accordance with state regulations. Proof of such inoculations and health records shall be kept on file in the pet registration roster found at the reception desk or in the office of the Director of the Activity Department.
   d. All visiting pet owners shall sign in at the reception desk in the pet registration roster at the beginning and end of each visit and are responsible for the pet's activities and behavior.
   e. All license and health records shall be updated annually — rabies every 3 years.
   f. Visiting dogs or cats shall not be in estrus.
   g. Visiting dogs or cats shall be housebroken if more than four month old. Younger dogs or cats may be admitted if kept in a box or basket suitable to contain any "accidents."

h. Visiting dogs shall be licensed and wear an identification tag on the collar or harness.

4. Residential Pets

a. A residential pet is defined as any animal that resides at the Masonic Home in excess of four hours during any calendar day. The financial responsibility for any residential pets shall be handled by the Activity Department.

b. All residential pets, except for fish, shall have a confinement area where they can be restricted from freely visiting with residents when appropriate. Fish shall be kept in aquariums throughout the Medical Center.

c. Pet care — The administrator is responsible for acceptable pet husbandry practices and may delegate specific duties to any other staff member except food handlers and staff involved in direct patient care. The areas of delegation shall include:

1. Food clean-up — handled by residents, supervised by the Activity Staff.

2. Waste clean-up — handled by Grounds staff.

3. Exercising — handled by residents, supervised by Activity Staff. Pets shall be permitted outside the facility only if under the supervision of a staff member or responsible person.

4. Grooming — handled by residents, supervised by Activity Staff. Pets shall be regularly groomed and receive a bath whenever indicated.

5. Bedding — handled by residents, supervised by Activity Staff. Pets shall be provided with a suitable bedding area. Bedding must be cleaned or changed as needed. Dirty bedding will be processed or disposed of as necessary.

d. Dogs and cats must be effectively housebroken. Animal waste shall be disposed of in a manner that prevents the material from becoming a community health or nuisance problem. Accepted methods include burial or disposal in sealed plastic bags. Municipally approved trash systems or the sewage system should be utilized for feces.

e. Proper and frequent hand-washing shall be a requirement of all persons handling any resident pet, its housing or any equipment associated with the pet.

f. The cooperating licensed veterinarian shall be Willingboro Veterinary Clinic, PA, Sidney Lane, Willingboro, NJ 08046 Tel. (609) 871-1600.

g. All pets must have current inoculations against the diseases particular to their species in accordance with State Regulations. Proof of such inoculations and health records shall be kept on file in the office of the Director of Activities.

h. Any pet found to be infested with external parasites (ticks, fleas or lice), or which vomits or has diarrhea must be removed immediately from the facility and taken to the cooperating licensed veterinarian. A newly completed NJ Animal Health Certificate shall be required before the animal can return to the facility.

i. The Burlington Township Health Department must be notified immediately by telephone of any pet which dies on the Home's premises. The body disposal must comply with the Burlington Township's ordinance.

Masonic Home Of New Jersey Visiting Pet Registration Sheet

(All information *must* be completed by pet owner.)

Name of Pet Owner_____

Telephone Number (___)_____-_____

Address_____

State _____ Zip Code_____

Pet Name_____

Description of Pet: Cat_____ Color_____ Breed_____

Dog_____ Color _____Breed_____ Weight_____

TDI Certification #_____

Temperament: Aggressive_____   Nervous_____

             Passive_____   Shy_____

To all pet therapy providers:
Please carefully read the statement on the following page and sign.
If your pet in any way does not conform to all standards included
in this statement, it may not visit in the building or anywhere on
the grounds of the Masonic Home of New Jersey. We appreciate
your cooperation in providing a part of our extensive pet therapy
program.

Sincerely,
Margaret N. Abdill, LPN, ADC
Director of Activities

Owner Statement:
As the owner of the above mentioned pet, I make the following statements. I have provided a health certificate signed by a licensed veterinarian indicating that this pet, if a dog, is up-to-date for all vaccinations against canine diseases of distemper, hepatitis, leptospirosis, parainfluenza, parvovirus, coronavirus, bordetella (kennel cough) and rabies. If my pet is a cat, proof of vaccination on a health certificate signed by a licensed veterinarian shall include feline pneumonitis, panleukopenia, rhinothracheitis, calicvirus, chlamydia and rabies. Any pet other than a cat or dog must have specific approval from the Director of the Activity Department. (Birds are not approved animals for pet therapy in this facility.) My pet is licensed in the town or city where I live. It is housebroken, well-groomed, free of any odor and is not infected with any external parasites such as ticks, fleas or lice. I will not bring my pet to this facility if it is in estrus (heat) or shows inappropriate signs of sexual behavior. I understand that my pet must remain on a leash at all times while in the facility or on the grounds and additionally be controlled by verbal commands. My pet has never shown inappropriate or aggressive behavior. I also understand that my pet may not be in areas where food is being served. As the owner of this pet I understand that I am liable and responsible for its behavior and activities while in this facility. Finally, I am aware that I must sign in and fill in the required information in the pet registration roster at the beginning and end of each visit.

Witness_____ Date ____/____/____

Signed_____ Date ____/____/____

Printed Name_____

Pet Owner Signature	Date	Time In	Time Out	Resident Visiting	Comments
1.					
2.					
3.					
4.					
5.					
6.					
7.					
8.					
9.					
10.					
11.					
12.					
13.					
14.					
15.					
16.					
17.					
18.					
19.					
20.					

Showing Appreciation to your Pet Therapy Providers

Saying "thank you" to those who may assist you in providing pet therapy is always a good idea, but expressing your gratitude by sending a letter or having a "special appreciation night" is going the extra mile. It demonstrates how much you appreciate the many hours your providers have given to training and grooming their pets and spending time in your facility.

I am most fortunate to have access to several sources which provide animals besides our facility pets for pet therapy sessions.

There is an animal farm not far from our facility whose staff makes visits with several animals at a time. Whenever they visit, we give them a donation of money to help them sustain their work.

Family and friends visit, bringing in their pets. On their first visit they are given a thank you letter (see example, below) with a small bag of dog treats attached. In addition, every June we have a "pet appreciation night" which everyone who has visited throughout the year is invited to attend.

We have a wonderful group of volunteers who come on a monthly basis from September to June. All these folks have had pets certified by Therapy Dogs International. They have been coming to the Home for many years and are very faithful to their commitment. It was actually for this group that our "pet appreciation night" was started.

We also have a volunteer who brings in her Dachshund, Ginger. She has accumulated over 500 hours of volunteer time!

And, of course, there are staff members who bring their pets in to visit.

Everyone who comes to the Home with a pet registers in our pet registry book and is invited to our "pet appreciation night." We have had different pet appreciation night programs each year, however we have always included the following:

1. A personal invitation sent by mail to each participant, requesting an RSVP.

2. A room set up with tables and chairs, the tables set with linens and decorated with baskets of "Doggie Bones."
3. An awards table which includes a framed certificate of appreciation from the Home. The provider's name is on the certificate, which is signed by our administrator and the chairman of the Board of Trustees.
4. A gift given with the presentation of each certificate. This may be a ceramic animal (made by our residents), pet shampoo or a package of homemade dog biscuits (made by our cooking class), along with a bone shaped cookie cutter, a copy of the recipe and a box of dog biscuits. Use your imagination — you never know what you may come up with.
5. A table of refreshments that usually includes a fruit punch, fresh fruit salad, tea sandwiches and bowls of potato chips.

Our "pet appreciation night" program has varied over the years. Some of the programs that have been presented include:

- A slide presentation of our facility years ago, showing the contrast with how it looks today.
- A speaker who trains dogs for the hearing impaired.
- A viewing of the television program AM Philadelphia. They had been at the Home and did a program on our pet therapy program.
- A video about companion dogs.

After the certificate and gifts are presented and the program is over, my staff and I usually serve the food. It's always a treat to be served on special occasions and everyone seems to enjoy it.

And sometimes there are great stories to share. One night I was standing near the refreshment table, speaking with a faithful volunteer who has come in regularly with her dog. As she spoke I noticed that her rather large but extremely well-behaved dog was paying particular attention to the fact that she was deeply involved in conversation and that the refreshment table was at nose level.

With one sudden graceful swoop, the dog inhaled about half of the sandwich tray and in an instant was again sitting regally as if nothing had happened. In view of the fact this lady felt so much pride in her dog's handsome appearance and his mastery of obedience — he was on a sit-stay command — I just winked at him, finished my conversation with his master and removed the tray from the table. He looked at me as if to say, "I understand that this will be our little secret."

Thank You Letter — Pet Provider's First Visit

Masonic Home of New Jersey
"We Prove We Care"

Dear Friend,

You are special and I would like to extend to you a particularly warm welcome and thanks for taking the time to bring your pet to our facility.

Pet therapy is a vital part of our extensive activity program here at the Masonic Home of New Jersey. We appreciate your efforts in training, grooming and keeping your pets healthy so that they will be appropriately readied to visit our residents.

We request your cooperation in filling out the pet registry book whenever you arrive for or depart from a visit. Supplying us with the necessary information regarding current shots and license numbers is also very much appreciated.

We hope your pet will enjoy the attached treat and that you will gain much satisfaction from the joy you bring to our special residents.

With much appreciation,

Margaret N. Abdill, LPN, ADC
Director of Activities

Sample Invitation To Pet Appreciation Night

Masonic Home of New Jersey
"We Prove We Care"

Dear Friends,

The Masonic Home of New Jersey is able to boast about its extensive activity programming and you have been a part of our success.

A review of our pet therapy registry shows that you have visited the Home with your pet, either with our regular pet therapy group or individually, visiting a specific family member or friend.

We would like to honor you for the time and effort you have given in preparing for and providing pet therapy. You and your pet are cordially invited to attend our pet appreciation night on Wednesday, May 6, 1992 at 7:00 P.M. in Grow Memorial Hall.

We hope you will be able to attend and leave with a feeling of pride in knowing you have assisted in enhancing the quality of life for the residents at our facility. Please RSVP to the Activity Department at 386-0300 ext. 212 no later than May 4, 1992.

We look forward to sharing this special evening with you.

Sincerely,

Margaret N. Abdill, LPN, ADC
Director of Activities

PS: This special invitation is also extended to owners of recently certified therapy dogs. You are invited to preview the facility and, if you desire, become one of our regular visitors.

Sample Follow-Up Thank You Letter

Masonic Home of New Jersey
"We Prove We Care"

May 24, 1993

Dear Friend,

We're very sorry you were unable to be with us on Wednesday, May 12th when we held our pet appreciation night. Enclosed is your certificate of appreciation for service to our Masonic Home residents.

Our residents, our Board of Trustees and especially our entire Activity Staff thank you for your contribution of time in providing pet therapy here at the Masonic Home. Each visit you make is a special time for our "animal lovers" who look forward with so much anticipation to the hours of companionship and joy you and your pet provide.

Please know that your attention and commitment to keeping the wonder of pets alive in the hearts of our Masonic Home family is appreciated and admired.

Sincerely,

Margaret N. Abdill, LPN, ADC
Director of Activities

Delta Society Pet Partners Program

Health Screening For Animals
Additional Temperament Tests

Described below are the additional "test situations" which must be performed before, during or immediately after the physical exam.

These tests are very important in ensuring the well-being of the animals who participate in visitation programs. They will help us assess how this animal might react to a frail elderly person, Alzheimer's patient, enthusiastic child and others. Please give us your honest assessment.

The tests screen for friendliness, socialization, docility and ability to react to startling stimuli without panic, with sensitivity and forgiveness and without aggression.

If an animal displays unacceptable behavior, we can suggest ways for the owner to work to change the behavior. Also, an animal may still be eligible to visit in specific situations even without "passing" certain tests.

Unacceptable behavior includes scratching, growling, snapping or biting people or other animals, jumping on people and nervous or aggressive behavior.

Directions for completing this evaluation: Mark the behaviors as Acceptable (A) or Unacceptable (U) and add a few comments as to "why" in the space provided. Thank you again for your assistance.

Note: All tests may be modified for large/farm animals.

1. A crowded waiting area with other animals (of varying species, if possible), various ages and gender of people (including children if possible).
   Number of people in waiting area: Male_____ Female_____
   Children_____ Teens_____ Adults_____ Elderly_____
   A_____ U_____ Why?_____

2. Reaction to strangers approaching: i.e.: children, men, women. (Circle)
   A_____ U_____ Why?_____

3. Person gesturing wildly: Someone in waiting room or entering room during examination.
   A_____ U_____ Why?_____

4. Loud unusual sounds: Person pushing IV pole/gurney/wheelchair toward pet.
   A_____ U_____ Why?_____

5. Loud/Unusual sounds: Someone drops stainless steel pan near animal (preferably out of eyesight).
   A_____ U_____ Why?_____

6. Sensitivity to touch: Observe during exam — especially handling of feet, webbing of toes, tail, mouth. Give animal a big hug, firm pats on head. Clip toenails (if needed and appropriate).
   A_____ U_____ Why?_____

7. Handling by others: Hand pet to others or have them hold pet for several minutes while owner moves away. (Large animals — hand lead to others, have them walk with animal away from you).
   A_____ U_____ Why?_____

8. Give animal a treat/tidbit — observe how they take it (i.e. politely).
   A_____ U_____ Why?_____

Additional comments/observations:
_____
_____
_____

References

Arkow, P. **How to Start a Pet Therapy Program: A Guideline for Health Care Professionals.** 37 Hillside Road, Stratford, NJ 08084.

Arkow, P. (Ed.) 1987. **Loving Bond: Companion Animals in the Helping Professions.** R&E Publications.

Bernard, S. 1988. "The Utilization Of Animals As A Therapeutic Modality." *Occupational Therapy Forum*, III(29), 1,3.

Best Martini, E., M. A. Weeks and P. Wirth. 1996. **Long Term Care for Activity and Social Service Professionals — Second Edition.** Ravensdale WA: Idyll Arbor, Inc.

Bredenberg, D. 1990, May. "Developing A Companion Animal Program." *Nursing Homes*, 21-29.

Budiansky, S. 1989, March 20. "The Ancient Contract." *US News and World Report*, 75-79.

Cutler Riddick, C. 1985. "Health, Aquariums and the non-institutionalized elderly." In M. Sussman (ed.), **Pets and the Family** (pp. 63-173). New York: Haworth Press.

Fox, M. W. 1992. **Understanding Your Dog: Everything You Want to Know About Your Dog But Haven't Been Able to Ask Him.** New York: St. Martins Press.

Fox, N. 1979. **How To Put Joy Into Geriatric Care.** Bend, OR: Geriatric Press, Inc.

Francis, G. 1984. "Plush Animals As Therapy In A Nursing Home." *Clinical Gerontologist*, 2(4), 75-76.

Francis, G. and A. Baly. 1986, May/June. "Plush Animals — Do They Make A Difference?" *Geriatric Nursing*, 140-142.

Francis, G. and B. Munjas. 1988, June. "Plush Animals and the Elderly." *The Journal of Applied Gerontology*, 7(2), 161-172.

George, J. C. 1985. **How to Talk to Your Animals.** Orlando, FL: Harcourt.

Gowing, C. 1984. **The effects of minimal care pets on homebound elderly and their professional caregivers.** Unpublished doctoral dissertation, University of Illinois at Urbana-Champaign.

Jackson, L. (Ed.). 1990. **The Value of Activities in Marketing.** Columbia, MO: Project Life, University of Missouri.

Katcher, A. H. 1982, September-October. "Are Companion Animals Good for your Health?" *Aging*, 2-8.

Koedel, F. B. and M. J. Brunecz. 1989. "Hello Dolly." *Occupational Therapy Forum*, IV(4), 1,3.

Lee, R. L. **Guidelines: Animals in Nursing Homes.** Renton, WA: The Delta Society.

Masonic Home of New Jersey,
1. The Masonic Home Story
2. Masonic Home Pet Policy — 3/96
3. Masonic Home Pet Registry Sign-In Sheet
4. Thank You Letter To Visitors Providing Pet Therapy
5. Fish Tank Instructions
6. King's Puppy Schedule
7. Name The Puppy Contest
8. Invitation to Pet Appreciation Night 1992
9. Follow-Up Letter For Pet Appreciation Night 1993

Meyer, N. 1984. **A Pet Owner's Guide to Dog Crate.** Copies Available from: Nicki Meyer Educational Effort, Inc., 31 Davis Hill Rd, Weston, CT 06883.

Meyer, N. 1984, May. "Dog Crates — Cruelty or Kindness?" *Dog Fancy*, 18-20.

Pechter, K. 1985, August. "Pet therapy for heart and soul." *Prevention*, 80-86.

Pet Food Institute. **Housing Happy Pets and Happy People: Management Guidelines.** Copies Available from: Pet Food Institute, 1101 Connecticut Ave. NW, Suite 700, Washington, DC 20036.

Schwartz, C. *Every Dog Needs a Number.* Brandy Lane Dog Training School, 135 Kings Road, Mt. Holly, NJ 08060.

Toufexis, A. 1987, March 30. "Furry and Feathery Therapists". *Time*, 74.

Viorst, J. 1971. **The Tenth Good Thing About Barney.** New York: Atheneum.

Wallace, J. E. and S. Naderman. 1987. *The Journal of Applied Gerontology*, 6(2), 183-188.

Vogel, B. 1984. **Pets and Their People**. Viking Press.

Appendix

There are a wealth of resources available on the topic of pet therapy. This list is organized by topic: first general resources are listed, then those dealing with specific therapy pets.

Books, magazines, newsletters and journals — all are great resources which can help you in gathering the information you need to start a program. They offer knowledge and often useful insights or tips about programs, pets, breeders, training and much more.

National organizations are another rich source of information on all topics of pets and pet therapy. They can also direct you to specific resources in your area. Some of these local resources are included here, for those interested in contacting them directly.

Keep in mind that new books and articles are always being published: this is only a partial list of resources that are available today. Check your local library for additional publications.

Many of us are becoming 'computer literate', and a remarkable number of organizations are now developing their own information pages on the World Wide Web, and/or can be reached via e-mail. We have included many e-mail addresses, as well as one web address which maintains extensive links for animal assisted therapy groups, as well as the "hard copy" information on these groups.

Finally, a list of pet supply catalogs is included.

Pet Therapy (General)

Books:

Arkow, Phil. **How to Start a Pet Therapy Program: A Guideline for Health Care Professionals**. 37 Hillside Road, Stratford, NJ 08084. Phone: 609-627-5118, fax 609-627-2252, e-mail, arkowpets@aol.com.

Cusack, Odean and Elaine Smith. 1984. **Pets And The Elderly: The Therapeutic Bond**. New York: Haworth Press.

Katcher, Aaron H. and Alan M. Beck (Eds.). **New Perspectives On Our Lives With Companion Animals**. Philadelphia: University of Pennsylvania Press.

Journal Articles:

American College of Health Care Administrators. 1984. "Pets and Patients: Therapy That Works." *The Journal of Long Term Care Administration*. 12(4); Winter.

Kits:

Bi-Folkal Productions. *Remembering Pets*. A complete multimedia, multi-sensory program kit of reminiscence resources on the topic of pets. For more information about that kit and 15 others, contact Bi-Folkal at 809 Williamson Street, Madison, WI 53703 (608) 251-2818.

Animal/Pet Therapy Information:

The Humane Society of the United States, 2100 L Street NW, Washington, DC 20037 (201) 452-1100.

Dogs

Books:

American Kennel Club. 1992. **The Complete Dog Book**. New York: Howell Book House.

Cohen, Barbara, and Louise Taylor. 1989. **Dogs & Their Women**. Little, Brown and Company.

Davis, Kathy D. 1992. **Therapy Dogs: Training Your Dog To Reach Others**. New York: Howell Book House Inc.

Denoff, Donald E., DVM with Emily West. **There Are No Bad Dogs**. Globe Communications Corp.

The Monks of New Skete. 1991. **The Art of Raising a Puppy**. Little, Brown and Company.

The Monks of New Skete. 1978. **How To Be Your Dog's Best Friend, A Training Manual For Dog Owners**. Little, Brown and Company.

Pepper, Jeffrey. 1984. **The Golden Retriever**. T.F.H. Publications, Inc.

Pryor, Karen. 1996. **Don't Shoot the Dog**. A Bantam New Age Book

Pryor, Karen. 1985 **How to Teach Your Dog to Play Frisbee**. New York: Simon and Schuster

Schwartz, Charlotte. 1984. **Friend To Friend**. New York: Howell Book House Inc.

Schwartz, Charlotte. 1987. **The Howell Book of Puppy Raising**. New York: Howell Book House Inc.

Tortora, Daniel F. 1983 **The Right Dog For You**. Fireside.

Walsh, James. E. Jr. 1988. **Golden Retriever**. T.F.H. Publications, Inc.

Woodhouse, Barbara. 1984. **No Bad Dogs — The Woodhouse Way**. New York: Summit Books.

Magazines:
Dog Fancy
Subscription Department
PO Box 53264
Boulder, CO 80323-3264

Dog World
PO Box 5384
Harlan, IA 51593-2884

Training Programs:
Brandy Lane Dog Training School
1162 King's Road
Mt. Holly, NJ 08060
(609) 261-1321

Cats

Magazines:
Cat Fancy
Subscription Department
PO Box 52864
Boulder, CO 80323-2864

Birds

Magazines:
Bird Talk
Subscription Department
PO Box 57347
Boulder, CO 80323-7347

Organizations

Finding a Group to Join: (This information — slightly amended — comes courtesy of Diane Blackman, of Dog-Play, Inc. The web page which contains it can be found on the Internet by typing: http://www.dog-play.com/join.html. This is part of a much larger site, a wonderful resource for dog-owners, which is accessed by typing: http://www.dog-play.com.)

Although a large number the groups listed here are involved in dog-assisted therapy, there are still quite a few that are more generalized, or who can point you in the direction of a group that specializes in your therapy animal.

If you are using a dog, then this list may be invaluable. Finding someone to certify your dog is often a frustrating experience. The evaluations offered by the national organizations aren't always as frequent and convenient as you might like. Many local organizations offer certification, at least as long as you visit under their program. Joining a local group can be a big help in getting you started. Here I hope to collect information that will be local to you. It will take some time and your participation. The list is organized by state.

National Organizations:

Therapy Dogs Inc.
PO Box 2786
Cheyenne, WY 82003
(307) 638-3223
Ann Butrick, Executive Director

Therapy Dogs International
719 Darla Lane
Fallbrook, CA 92028-1505
e-mail to Therapy Dogs International
tdi@gti.net

Delta Society Pet Partners Programs
289 Perimeter Rd. East
Renton, WA. 98055
(800) 869-6898 (voice)
(425) 235-1076 (fax)
e-mail:
deltasociety@cis.compuserve.com

Love on a Leash
3809 Plaza Dr. #107-309
Oceanside, CA 92056
(619) 630-4824
Liz Palika, President —
watachie@aol.com
Christina Sahhar, Membership
Chairman — christie@cts.com

Local Organizations:

ARIZONA

Companion Animal Association of
Arizona
Box 5006
Scottsdale, AZ 85261-5006
(602) 258-3306

Tucson Animal Assisted
Psychotherapy Associates, Inc.
(520) 744-9037
{Not dogs, horses!}

CALIFORNIA

Latham Foundation
Latham Plaza Bldg.
Clement & Shiller Streets
Alameda, California 94501
e-mail to Latham Foundation:
lathm@aol.com
(510) 521-0920

Marin Humane Society
171 Bel Marin Keys Blvd.
Novato, CA 94949
(415) 883-4621 (Voice)
(415) 382-1349 (Fax)
e-mail: marinhs@petnet.net

Friendship Foundation
PO Box 6525
Albany, CA 94706
(510) 528-9104
contact person: Elizabeth Soares
Friendship Foundation volunteers and
their pets visit various health care
facilities to enrich the lives of children
and adults. A designated liaison
arranges and attends all visits. Pets are
required to undergo complete health
exams and temperament testing.

S*M*A*R*T* Dogs, Inc.
55 Cambrian Avenue
Piedmont, California 94611

Therapy Pets
PO Box 32288
Oakland, California 94604

San Francisco SPCA
2500 16th Street
San Francisco, CA
(415) 554-3000
e-mail: public_info@sfspca.org

PAWS — Pets are Wonderful Support
PO Box 460489
San Francisco, CA 94146-0489
(415) 824-4040

Furry Friends Foundation
Pet Assisted Therapy Services
PO Box 90550, San Jose, CA 95109
e-mail to PATS:
info@furryfriends.org
(408) 280-6171

Pet-Helpers Humane Society of
Sonoma County
Pet-Helpers
442 Steele Lane
Santa Rosa, CA 95403-3149
melinda@bikepro.com
(408) 542-0882 extension 207
(Jennifer)

Assistance Dog Institute
PO Box 2334
Rohnert Park, CA 94927
(707) 762-5607

Santa Barbara Humane Society
5399 Overpass Road
Santa Barbara, CA 93111
sos@west.net
(805) 964-4777

"Create-A-Smile" Animal-Assisted-
Therapy Team LA
1140 Westwood Blvd. Suite #205
Los Angeles, CA 90024
(310) 208-3631 Voice
(310) 208-2779 Fax
website: www.aat.org
e-mail: therapy@aat.org

Therapy Dogs: Our Best Friends
Therapy Dog Program, Inc.
PO Box 2345
Spring Valley, CA 91979

COLORADO

HSBV DeTails:
Lending a Helping Paw
The Humane Society of Boulder
Valley
2323 55th Street
Boulder, CO 80301
(303) 442-4030

CONNECTICUT

Tails of Joy, TDI
Janet Miller, Director (also TDI
Evaluator)
PO Box 187
Pleasant Valley, CT 06063
Contact: Jan Miller
e-mail: tabrac@esslink.com

FLORIDA

The ComForT Program (Companions
For Therapy)
c/o the Area Agency on Aging
2639 North Monroe Street
Suite 145B
Tallahassee, FL 32302
Contact: Julia Osmond
jposmond@nettally.com

ILLINOIS

Rainbow Animal-Assisted Therapy
PO Box 531
Northbrook IL 60065-0531
(312) 283-1129
Nancy Lind, President

PAN: People, Animals, Nature
Coalition of Chicago Area Animal-
Assisted Therapy Human Service
Providers
1820 Princeton Circle
Naperville IL 60565
(708) 369-8328
President: Debbie Coultis

Encouraging Word Animal-Assisted
Therapy
Mary Jacobs, Licensed Clinical
Professional Counselor
Certified School Psychologist
Animal-Assisted Therapy Programs
e-mail: u45301@uicvm.uic.edu

Tree House Animal Foundation
(312) 784-5605 (voice)
(312) 784-2332 (fax)
e-mail: treehouse@tezcat.com

MARYLAND

Pets on Wheels
2619 Maryland Ave.
Baltimore, MD 21218
(410) 366-7387

Fidos for Freedom, Inc.
PO Box 5508
Laurel, MD 20726

MASSACHUSETTS

Pets and People Foundation
11 Apple Crest Road
Weston, MA 02193
(617) 899-5029

MINNESOTA

Bark Avenue on Parade, Inc.
PO Box 62112
Minneapolis, MN 55426
e-mail: bouvweb@sprynet.com

Elk River Therapy Dogs
Elk River, Minnesota
e-mail to Lori
woof1@worldnet.att.net

MISSOURI

Support Dogs, Inc.
3958 Union Rd.
St. Louis, MO 63125
(314) 892-2554
contact person: Chris Curtis or
e-mail Mary D: Luvtrooper@aol.com

NEW HAMPSHIRE

New Hampshire SPCA
PO Box 196 Route 108
Stratham, NH 03885
(603) 772-2921

NEW JERSEY

Therapy Dogs International, Inc.
6 Hilltop Road
Mendham, NJ 07945
(201) 543-0888
fax (201) 543-0989
e-mail tdi@gti.net

NEW MEXICO

Southwest Canine Corps of
Volunteers
PO Box 14967
Albuquerque, NM 87191
e-mail to: sheryll@rapunzel.unm.edu
(Sheryll Barker)
e-mail to: dmiller@nmia.com
e-mail to: vangul@nmia.com

Los Alamos Caring Canine
Companions
924 Tewa Loop
Los Alamos, NM 87544
(505) 661-9619
Contact Lynn Wysocki-Smith

NEW YORK

Pet Assisted Therapy Facilitation
Certificate Program
State University of New York
(401) 463-5809

OREGON

Welcome Waggers Therapy Dogs
22830 Alsea Hwy.
Philomath, OR 97370
(541) 929-5064
e-mail: malpals@peak.org

OKLAHOMA

Petworks In Progress Foundation
PO Box 6282
Norman, OK 73070-6282
(405) 364-1525
e-mail outanorm@inetnow.com
Kris Butler, President, Petworks in
Progress Foundation

OHIO

Prescription: Dog Love
Mentor Contact: Lynn Schaber
e-mail: Lynn.Schaber@alltel.com
Akron, Ohio

PENNSYLVANIA

Lehigh Valley K-9 Therapy
Association, Chapter 100
42 MacIntosh Dr.
Easton, PA 18045
(610) 559-7071
e-mail: xracers@prolog.net
John McMurray, Director, TDI
Evaluator for the Lehigh Valley area

K's K-9 Therapy Dog Group
4 Sycamore Circle
Lititz, PA 17543-8744
(717) 627-3586
Contact: Kay Melchi

Lebanon County Kennel Club
Sally Henry (contact person)
(717) 273-8612

TEXAS

Paws Across Texas
4413 Thrasher Ct.
Ft. Worth, TX 76137
Virginia Hyatt, President
(817) 577-1103
e-mail: angiem@airmail.net

Therapy Pet Pals of Texas
3930 Bee Caves Road, Suite 6-B
Austin, TX 78746
(512) 347-1984

Paws for Caring
740 Mulberry
Bellaire, TX 77401
(713) 667-8114
Facilities Volunteer Coordinator:
Melinda Ashman (713) 995-1378

Animal Outreach
Brazos Animal Shelter
2207 Finfeather Road
Bryan, Texas 77801
(409) 775-5755

UTAH

The Good Shepherd Association
PO Box 650
Riverton, UT 84065
(801) 253.1900
(801) 253.4900 (Fax)
e-mail TGSA: goodshep@aros.net

WASHINGTON

Kitsap Humane Society
9167 Dickey Road NW
Silverdale, WA 98383
(360) 692-6977

People Pet Partnership
Charlene Douglas, Assistant Director
College of Veterinary Medicine
Washington State University
Pullman, WA 99164-7010
(509) 335-1303
(509) 335-4569

CANADA

St. John Ambulance Therapy Dog
Program
1199 Deyell 3rd Line
Milbrook, Ontario L0A 1G0

Copyright © 1996, Diane Blackman
Contact DOG-PLAY at: webmaster@dog-play.com

PUBLICATIONS: Payment of a small membership fee to the
organization is usually required in order to receive these.

Alpha Bits
Alpha Affiliates, Inc.
103 Washington Street, Suite 362
Morristown, NJ 07960

Therapy Dogs International
Ursula Kempe, Treasurer
260 Fox Chase Road
Chester, NJ 07930

Canine Hearing Companions Inc.
247 E Forrest Grove Road
Vineland, NJ 08360
Phone: (609) 696-0969

The Seeing Eye Guide
PO Box 375
Morristown, NJ 07963-0375
Phone: (201) 539-4425

The Clapper Independence Dogs Inc.
146 State Line Road
Chadds Ford, PA 19317
Phone: (215) 358-2723

Canine Companions For
Independence National Office
PO Box 446
Santa Rosa, CA 95420-0446
Phone: (707) 528-0830

Interaction, A Delta Society
Publication
289 Perimeter Road East
Renton, WA 98055-1329
(800) 869-6898

The Latham Letter
Latham Plaza Building
Clement and Schiller Street
Alameda, CA 94501
Phone: (510) 521-0920
Fax: (510) 521-9861

Pet Supply Catalogs

Discount Master Animal Care
Division of Humboldt Industries, Inc.
Lake Road, PO Box 3333
Mountaintop, PA 18707-0330
Phone: (800) 346-0749

The Dog's Outfitter
Division of Humboldt Industries, Inc.
1 Maplewood Drive
PO Box 2010
Hazelton, PA 18201-0676

Pedigrees
1989 Transit Way
Box 905
Brockport, NY 14420-0905
Phone: (716) 673-1431

J-B Wholesale Pet Supplies, Inc.
289 Wagaraw Road
Hawthorne, NJ 07506
Phone: (800) 526-0388
In New Jersey: (201) 423-2222
Fax: (201) 423-1181

Drs. Foster & Smith, Inc.
2253 Air Park Road
PO Box 100
Rhinelander, WI 54501-0100
Phone: (800) 826-7206

R. C. Steele
1989 Transit Way
Box 910
Brockport, NJ 14420-0910
Phone: (800) 872-3773

About The Authors

Margaret N. Abdill, LPN, ADC worked for many years in obstetrical nursing, assisting women through the stages of pregnancy and the experience of childbirth and teaching new mothers to care for their infants. This was the fulfillment of a childhood dream to be a nurse. However, a career change took her into gerontology nursing, which then opened the door into the field of activity programming.

Since entering the field, Margaret has worked to advance it as a profession in the state of New Jersey. She was a charter member of the New Jersey Activity Professionals' Association, assisting in the creation of the organization. She has served for many years as the registration chair for Spring Workshops and Annual Conventions. She has also held the office of Treasurer of the organization for five years and is currently serving as President..

Margaret has also served her local organization, the Tri-County Activity Coordinators Association, as Treasurer, Secretary and President.

She is the Director of Activities at the Masonic Home of New Jersey, a 517 bed facility. Since taking over the department at the end of 1985, she has greatly increased resident participation and has been a motivating force in the introduction of progressive and innovative activity programming there. She was a vital part of the committee which started a Special Care Unit. She continues to work closely with the Director of Nursing, Marjorie Berleth, MSHA, RNC to maintain its success and meet the on-going needs of all their residents.

Margaret is an active member of her church as well as several women's organizations where she has held local and state offices. In her leisure time she enjoys baking, singing in her church choir, playing the piano, embroidery and sewing. Most of all she enjoys caring for her "boys": King, Bandit, Prancer and Nicky. But she admits she could not do it all without the love and support from her husband, Firman.

Her hope in putting together this manual is that readers will be encouraged to start a pet therapy program that suits their needs and provides a more home-like atmosphere for the residents that they serve.

Harriet Ciccotosto has been in the field of activities for over ten years, the last two and a half of which have been as Activity Director at the Baptist Home of South Jersey in Riverton, New Jersey. She is very active in her profession, having held many offices (including president) in her local activity association and served on the founding committee of the state activity association (NJAPA). She is currently on the Resource Review Committee of the National Association of Activity Professionals (NAAP).

Ms. Ciccotosto has a BA degree in music from Combs College in Germantown, Pennsylvania, is certified as a consultant by the National Certification Council for Activity Professionals and was listed in *Who's Who of American Professional Women* in 1990. She is on the Burlington County Boards of the American Cancer Society and Directors of Volunteers in Associations (DOVIA).

Randie Dale Duretz, ADC, is the Activity Director at Luther Woods Convalescent Center in Hatboro, Pennsylvania, where she works with both young adults and senior citizens who are convalescent, rehabilitation and head injury residents. She has also passed the Remotivation Therapy Course and in her spare time takes prize-winning photographs and works closely with law firms. Ms. Duretz is the proud owner of three lovable, friendly, obedient, certified therapy dogs — rough collies who are "Lassie look-a-likes."

Lynne Martin Erickson is one of the co-founders (along with Kathryn Leide) of Bi-Folkal Productions, Inc., a non-profit organization created to provide older adults with opportunities for remembering their lives.

Pat Gonser, a registered nurse, became interested in animal therapy while attending Texas Woman's University, Denton, Texas where she earned a Doctor of Philosophy in Nursing in 1988. Following a move to Buffalo, NY she began raising and breeding cats specifically for temperament and companionability in therapy programs. She was at the time an Assistant Professor of Nursing at D'Youville College, Buffalo, NY, was a member of Delta Society's Pet Partners Program and the network coordinator for the Western New York Network Group of the Delta Society. She also co-founded Positively Unique Fur Friends.

Denise Juppé has a BA in Zoology from Duke University and has spent much of her career in software development. She has always maintained a parallel interest in writing, participating in a writers' group in Acton, MA for several years. She spent the last three years in Belgium; on her return to the US she began working as a freelance editor for Idyll Arbor, Inc. Ms. Juppé lives with a small menagerie (a dog, two cats, two children and a husband) in Issaquah, WA.

Lori Kilburn, a recreational therapist, graduated from Mediaville College in 1985. She has a long-standing interest in animals, having assisted in the foundation of the Rivendell Recreational Horseback Riding Program in 1982. Ms. Kilburn has served on the Board of Directors of Rivendell and has been an instructor in their riding program. She is a member of Delta Society's Pet Partners Program and co-founded of Positively Unique Fur Friends.

Charlotte Schwartz founded Brandy Lane Dog Training School. She was the owner for approximately 20 years and retired in 1986.

Lloyd A. Taylor is a retired minister who lives in a retirement complex in Edmond, Oklahoma.

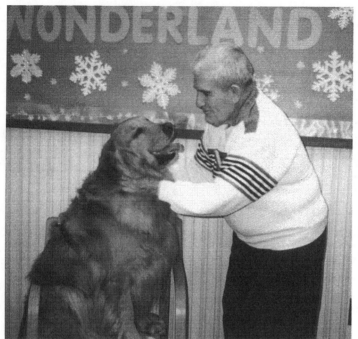

Bill Richmond enjoys a few moments with Nickie as he makes visits in the Medical Center

Index

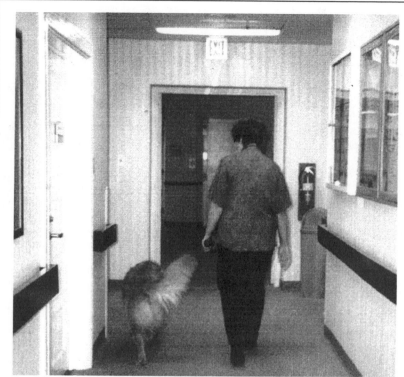

Pat Mitchell returns to the woodshop with Nickie after a pet therapy session in the Medical Center.